Perspective of the Reproductive Health in Manipur

Dr. Pebam Krishnakumari

AKANSHA PUBLISHING HOUSE

4649-B/21, Ansari Road, Darya Ganj, New Delhi-110 002 (India)

AKANSHA PUBLISHING HOUSE
4649-B/21, Ansari Road,
Darya Ganj, New Delhi-110 002
Phones : 011-23263193, 09435116718
E-mail : ektabooks@yahoo.com
visit us : www.akanshapublishinghouse.com

Perspective of the Repruductive Health in Manipur

First Published : 2012

Reprint 2026

ISBN 978-81-8370-305-5

Published by Akansha Publishing House, New Delhi - 110002.

PRINTED IN INDIA

Contents

Acknowledgement

The scintilla of writing on Perspective on the **Reproductive Health of Women in Manipur** was instilled in me by Prof. P.C. Joshi, Department of Anthropology, University of Delhi. It is my privilege to convey a heartfelt sense of gratitude and highest veneration for his instrumentality in not only undertaking the theme but also for shaping it from time to time by valuable suggestions, useful ideas and laconic academic exchanges. No words of gratitude would be adequate to express the profound sense of indebtedness that I owe to Prof. P.C. Joshi. I bow down my head before his profound insight and unfathomable wisdom in the field of Medical Anthropology.

In no words, I can express my heartfelt thanks and profound sense of gratitude to Dr. M. Meghachandra Singh, Department of Community Medicine, Maulana Azad Medical College, New Delhi, particularly his great support and valuable suggestions. The time he spared in spite of his busy schedule to introduce me to the finer nuances of the subject and the different insights he offered has helped me in bringing this work to a satisfactory level.

I extend my heartfelt gratitude to Asst. Prof. M.C. Arunkumar, University of Manipur, for his invaluable comments, encouraging words and kind co-operation. Without his constant inspiration and guidance this book would not have seen the light of day. I also wish to express my gratitude to Dr. Manibabu for providing me with the necessary documents.

Special thanks to Dr.Angom Jyotsana,Gyneacologist (RIMS) for her indefatigable presence and her excellent clinical skills. Without her the clinical study would not have been possible. I also owe a debt of thanks to Dr. Mamta, Dr. Y. Ajitkumar, Dr. Supongmeren, Dr. Lalbiakdiki, Dr. Mark

Keyho and Dr. Tomar Basher for their hard work and enthusiasm in all the health camps.

I extend my gratitude to Dr. R.K. Sharan, Associate Professor, Department of Pathology, G.B. Pant Hospital, Indraprastha, New Delhi for conducting the entire laboratory test. This study would have remained incomplete without his help and co-operation.

I am also grateful to the Indian Council of Social Science Research (ICSSR) for granting me the fellowship for my research work. Without this fellowship this research work would have faced financial constraint.

I acknowledge a deep sense of gratitude for the emotional, intellectual and co-operative affinity of all those who manifestly or furtively contributed in accomplishing my work. I have been immensely helped by the people of Andro and Kwakeithel. I am indebted to them for their love and co-operation. Warm thanks to Thaba who accompanied me throughout my field work in Andro, without caring about foul weather conditions. Thanks to Hamlet, Sandhya, Memcha, Laibi, Dr Mani, Hemswori, Monsori, Shanti, Binasakhi, Kiranbala, Sobita, Kennedy, Somananda, Vinod and Umeshor who offered me generous hospitality and brightened up many moments in the field.without them this work would have been an impossible task. Thanks to Pebam Lolit who was more than eager to help me out in organizing the health camp in Kwakeithel.

I am indebted to Chaoba Heikrujam and Heikrujam Ongbi Nongalei for being the perfect host and for their affection and hospitality during my stay in Andro.

Thanks to Khomdram Premkumar and Khomdram Subhashchandra for their painstaking indefatigable efforts in going through the manuscript to avoid grammatical errors and pruninge out many crudities of style and diction.

I wish to express my gratitude to my parents, brother and sister for always having confidence in me, encouraging me to pursue my interest and for their unstinting support throughout.

Dr. Pebam Krishnakumari

Foreword

Medical science is a continuously advancing science. Research is the foundation of all the advances made in this field. The work done by Dr. Pebam Krishnakumari is remarkable. Her in-depth study of illness among rural/semi-urban womenfolk of Manipur—women who are less exposed to such researches—is truly commendable.

Women in general (and that of the lower strata of the society in particular) shy off from relating their sufferings and seek treatment only in the advanced stage of diseases. This proves challenging to the censured medical personnel.

It is the habit of women, who are less informed, to suffer quietly in the belief that it is "normal." They are reluctant to be physically examined and share intimate details about their problems. Therefore, it is imperative for the medical personnel to observe the body language and read between the lines when these women express their medical problems.

This study by Dr. Pebam Krishnakumari goes into the depth of illness in women, their body language and way of expressing half-hidden complaints and co-relates all these with the pathological findings to clinch the final, near-correct diagnosis.

Management of women illness in the reproductive age group in a better way will not only improve the health of women, but also help in bringing down the high infant mortality rate that India is facing right now.

Dr. Pebam Krishnakumari's research will facilitate the Ministry of Health and Family Welfare in formulating a long-term plan in safeguarding maternal and child welfare. It will be of great help if the curriculum in medical colleges includes the psychological aspects of women's way of expressing their gynecological problems.

S. Chaobi Devi

Dr. Mrs. S. Chaobi Devi
Retired Consultant (Obs & Gynae)
and HOD Dr. Ram Manohar Lohia Hospital.
New Delhi

Preface

Health of women in general and reproductive health in particular remains a largely unexplored area owing to the low priority attached to it. However, with the Cairo Conference in 1994 and Beyond Beijing in 1995, reproductive health of women came to the limelight. At the same time there is growing awareness about the scarcity of information concerning this issue. While there is a plethora of information on family planning and maternal health, which are referred to as "tip of the iceberg" concerning reproductive health, the magnitude of "the base of the iceberg" is not known and till now very little is known about reproductive morbidity and the underlying causes influencing women's health. This book endeavors to fill an important gap and describe the results of a study of reproductive morbidity in Manipur.

The main objectives of this study was to find out the magnitude of RTI's; to explore women's perception of their bodies, reproductive illnesses and health-seeking behavior; to compare women's reported symptoms with clinical examination and laboratory test results; to assess factors influencing the risks of RTI's including : personal, social, cultural, demographic, obstetric, reproductive history, use of contraception and hygiene, to compare the differences in reproductive health morbidity, differences in health-seeking patterns and risk factors of RTI's in Andro with that in kwakeithel. Another main objective of this study was to provide a basis for recommendation to health and family planning programmes.This study was a collaborative, integrated and inter-disciplinary dialogue between Medical Anthropology and Epidemiology, in terms of the methodology, to study the reproductive health of women in Manipur.

This book encapsulates: women's perception about their body anatomy and physiology and the practices they follow in accordance with these perceptions, women's perception of their respective illnesses in terms of aetiology and the terminology women used to describe illnesses. It also presents an ethnomedical model of "women's illness" along with the treatment-seeking behaviour.Women's self-reported symptoms, the prevalence of the three selected reproductive morbidities for this study and a comparison of reported symptom and clinically diagnosed condition is also presented. It also covers the risk factors of reproductive tract infections and prolapse in Andro and Kwakeithel.

This book also discusses the various entry points through which a meaningful and relevant reproductive health strategy could be developed in rural Andro and peri-urban Kwakeithel.

Dr. Pebam Krishnakumari

List of Abbreviations

AIDS	Acquired Immune Deficiency Syndrome
ANM	Auxiliary Nurse Midwives
CHC	Community Health Centre
EM	Explanatory Model
HIV	Human Immunodeficiency Virus
ICPD	International Conference on Population and Development
IIPS	Indian Institute of Population Science
IUD	Intra Uterine Device
LRTI	Lower Reproductive Tract Infection
MACS	Manipur state AIDS Control Organisation
MAMC	Maulana Azad Medical College, New Delhi
MoHFW	Ministry of Health and Family Welfare
NACO	National AIDS Control Organisation
NGO	Non-Government Organisation
NPV	Negative Predictive Value
PHC	Primary Health Centre
PID	Pelvic Inflammatory Disease
PPV	Positive Predictive Value
RHU	Rural Health Unit
RIMS	Regional Institute of Medical Sciences Manipur
RH	Reproductive Health

RM	Reproductive Morbidity
RTI	Reproductive Tract Infections
SPSS	Statistica Package for Social Science Research
STD	Sexually Transmitted Disease
STI	Sexually transmitted Infections
TBA	Traditional Birth Attendant
UN	United Nations
UNILO	United Nations International Labour Organisation
WCW	World Conference for Women
WHO	World Health Organisation

Local Terminology

Andro	A place of Schedule Caste Meitei community of Imphal East district Manipur
Kwakeithel	A place of populated Meitei community of Imphal West district Manipur
Maibi	A female birth attendant/midwife
Nisha Band	Women group/association
Meira Paibi	Women torch bearers
Meitei-lon	Meitei community language/dialect
Leikai	Locality
Leikai's	Localities
Phingou Chatpa	Vaginal discharge
Mangba	Menstruation
Mari Leinaba	Related
Anaba	Diesease
Angangkhao	Womb
Nanthaba	Prolapse
Loishang	Residing place of the deity Panam Ningthou
Pana	An institution in Andro
Ningthou	King
Sanamahi	Local religion
Lainingthou	Local/household deity

Khullakpa	Village chief
Luklakpa-	
Khujahanba-	
Pakhanglakpa-	***kind of various post of Andro***
Khabamlakpa-	
Yupanba-	
Kurak lamdaiba	A festival to prevent cattle epidemic
Khunthong lakpa	A sacrifice ceremony
Laisa tanba	A hunting festival by male bachelor
Saroi yenba	distribution of the cooked meat after hunting (a festival in Andro)
Thasi lubak	worshipping of sun and moon on every new moon
Laman chak pijaba	A ceremony offering food by sisters to their brothers
Cheiraoba	Meitei New Year
Sajibu	April month
Sougrakpa	Nobleman
Lai-haraoba	A festival to appease local deities
Saroi khangba	A ceremony to ward off evil spirits
Phanek	A woman wrap round common dress
Loi	Caste
Thagi khongkap lakpa	Monthly menstruation cycle
Lei-lakpa	A sign of maturity (blooming of flower)
Leisabi	A young unmarried girl
Pakholoi	A messenger
Koso	Dormitory
Puk-naba	Abdomen pain
Ethan thangatpa	feeling bloated up
Khwang naba	Back pain

E-nouba	A post-partum period
Nupa mangba	Male polluted
Mahik	Reference given to male Sperm (actually means germ)
Angang pokpa	Child birth
Mangba	Polluted/untouchable
Khoichum Leikham	Cultic Herb
Mayoknabi	One facing each other
Naopham	Placenta
Maiba	Male traditional healer
Kangkhil maru	A thing to throw and play the game of kang
Toubak/Wakthou	a kind of bamboo slice
Khangra mana	Leaf of Khangra tree
Esaiphu	Water pot
Tairen mana	Leaf of sacred Tairen tree
Pungphai	A kind of grass
E-manai	Remnant blood
Yu-machin	A pure local brew
Khwangchet punba	Abodominal binding tightly by a cloth
Kamuk	Rice cooked specially for mother in earthen pot
Nupigi anaba	Women's illness
Mantras	Sacred slokas
Puk suba	Massaging of abdomen
Khatpa	Implying sexual intercourse
Manam namthiba	Foul Smell
Manam namdaba	Odourless
Kangphan ekaithabi-	
Leiri-	a medicinal herb found locally used for treating women's illness

Ketuki-	
Komprek-	
Lai peruk-	
Sitamishri	Crystal sugar
Morok	Chilli
Yu	Local brew
Miron lietaba	Lack of helping hand
Hakchang mapan	
-thokpa	Prolapsed

1
Introduction

Reproductive health of women is an indispensable ingredient of human and a major determinant of human development. It affects everybody and involves intimate and highly valued aspects of life. Reproductive health is a fundamental human right. However, basic reproductive services have largely remained underserved or unserved for most of the poor sections of the populations of the developing world. Ensuring a healthy reproductive health is therefore, everyone's right and everyone's responsibility.

Reproductive Health Definition:

World Health Organization defines, "Reproductive health as a state of complete physical, mental and social well being and not merely the absence of disease or infirmity, in all matters relating to the reproductive system and to its functions and processes. Reproduction health therefore implies that people are able to have a satisfying and safe sex life, and that they have the caliber to reproduce and the freedom to decide it, when and how to do so. It also encapsulates sexual health and not merely counseling and care related to reproduction and sexually transmitted diseases".

(United Nations, 1994, Paragraph 7.2).

1.1 RESPONSIBILITY-CUM-JEOPARDY

From time immemorial, the duty of reproduction is assigned to women and as often in conjunction with disastrous health consequence of that assignment. Women may consider the ability to bear children to be the source of status in her life, her key to economic survival, the origin of her power on her family and society and a source of deep emotional satisfaction. She may also see it as the root cause of her oppression, a barrier to her participation's in the affairs of her community, an obstacle to personal fulfillment as well as the cause of intense pain and anxiety. However, the visualization of her reproductive caliber at any given moment in her life is for almost every woman an intimate, basic part of her physical existence and her sense of self, complemented with an often disastrous health consequence. There is always risk of disease or bodily harm that can be culminated from sex, pregnancy, childbirth and the means used to facilitate, prevent or control them. Illness and deaths from complications of pregnancy, childbirth, unsafe abortion, diseases of the reproductive tract and the improper use of contraceptive method tops the list of reproductive health threats to women worldwide (Jacobson, 1991; United Nations, 1995; WHO, 1995). As a Medical Anthropologist, our sole goal is to ensure a greater degree of health security of women by exploring out the handicaps and disabilities of women in a society enabling a woman to take up their responsibility *sans* jeopardy.

1.2 Factors contributing to reproductive morbidity

Reproductive health problems cannot be universally defined precisely because they require the local elaboration of meaning within particular cultural context. However, the unanimous surmization is that there is a complex interplay of socio-economic, environmental and cultural factors that contribute to reproductive morbidity particularly among women in developing countries. Poverty, ignorance, literacy and malnutrition are major determinant of women's health status. Also significant are the age at marriage and pregnancy, the number and frequency of child bearing and the number of unwanted pregnancies and abortions that contribute to morbidity and mortality among women and their babies. Another important factor is the health service related factors such as lack of access to quality reproductive health services. Biological as well as social factors affect women's health throughout their lives and have cumulative effect. Public health researchers suggest that social, political and structural factors must be addressed if reproductive health outcomes are to be improved (Bird and Bauman, 1995).

1.2.1 Determinants Fostering Reproductive Morbidity:

There are certain determinants which foster reproductive morbidity of women like taboo and poverty. On one hand, tabooed discussion on sex and sex related activity constraint women in opening up and express them to share their problems. On the other hand, in their daily struggle to meet the basic necessity of life they cannot avail the reproductive health facilities.

Taboo: An amazing thing about India where Kamasutra exist espousing liberal sex, talking openly about sex and desire remains a taboo in many cultural contexts. Often the language of sex is an area of contention. Words about sexual parts of the body or sexual activity may be totally unacceptable to older member of the same community. Taboo and silence limits the possibility of opening spaces for people to be able to express themselves and share their experience. Sex education in India has become a mission impossible. Women bear the brunt in silence and obscure the pain and suffering because of fear of social repercussion and stigma attached to it. The reproductive health needs are culture specific and pose implicit difficulties in their understanding because of inherent inhibitions, stigma and shame in Indian context. The traditional ideal of a women who is a virgin at marriage and is always faithful to her husband along with double standards that tacitly permit men to have pre-marital as well as extra marital sex had led to a situation where the existence of sex outside marriage is so well camouflaged as to be virtually invisible and definitely not discussed or acknowledged. Thus, the concept of sexuality of unmarried females adequately remains unexplored. Although there is a gross lack of information on sexual behaviour, Reproductive health concerns have legitimizes sexuality as an important concern and recognizes that men and women have sexual needs which must be addressed. It provides a sense of credibility to research on sexually related issues.

Poverty: In every society, women provide critical economic support to their families, alone or in conjunction with spouses by earning income in agriculture, in informal and formal labour markets. The notion that females do not contribute to family income is a tragic fallacy.Nearly 67 percent of India's economy is based on agriculture. Few resources reach women, although they comprise a large share of both paid and unpaid (family) agricultural labor (Chatterjee, 1991; Bennett, 1989). National survey data on which investment decision are based imply women make up 46 percent of the agricultural labor force (Chatterjee, 1991; Bennett, 1989). A study by the United Nation International Labor Organization detailing with the way rural women spent their time indicates that up to 90 percent of the rural women in India participate in agriculture (Chatterjee, 1991). However their contribution in economic front remains obscure making them invisible workforce. The hazardous endeavor undertaken by women to make both ends meet endangers their health in many ways. Poverty pressurizes both rural women as well as their urban counterparts to work through final stage of pregnancy, putting enormous demand on their physical energy and allowing to take little rest. The lifelong drain on physical stamina complicates the health of women.

In India, women work an average of 12-18 hours per day in their multiple roles with family as caretakers, educators, health promoters and income earners (Agarwal et al., 1990). Women engaged in a daily struggle to meet the basic needs cannot avail themselves of preventive health care for the exigencies of the unexpected illness.

1.3 EPIDEMIOLOGY AND MEDICAL ANTHROPOLOGY

This study will be a collaborative, integrated and interdisciplinary dialogue of Epidemiology and Medical Anthropology in terms of the methodology that will follow to study the reproductive health of women. Here both the discipline will be discussed - epidemiology and medical anthropology are scientific disciplines that search for patterns of disease and behaviour. They both have humanism at their core. However, tradition and history separate these two disciplines. Epidemiology tends to be statistical and quantitative while anthropology being largely textual and qualitative. To begin, epidemiology is derived from the Greek word *epi* meaning "upon" *demos* meaning "the populace or common people" and *logos* meaning "word". Epidemiology is literally the study of what is upon the populace, referring specifically to the burden of disease. But epidemiology is more than the study of epidemics. It is more conventionally defined as the study of the distribution and determinants of disease in human population. It focuses on population using statistics and probabilities. When epidemiologists work across different countries and within diverse groups in a single country they inevitably come into contact with cultural differences but culture is less widely appreciated in the epidemiological worldview. Epidemiology focuses on disease classification, prevalence, incidence, risk and behaviour in addition to other variable such as income, education, marital status, occupation, etc.

Medical anthropology also looks out for patterns but they find them in culturally conditioned responses to disease. Medical anthropologist studies the afflictions facing humankind and how human groups organize themselves to treat and explain the causes of suffering. They analyze the experiences and interpretations of healing, illness and determinants of disease. Culture influence the patterning of disease through many pathways, ranging from who is counted to what is noticed to where people obtain help for suffering.

As reproductive health problem is not just a biological problem but has a socio -cultural component a multi disciplinary approach is essential.

1.4 REPRODUCTIVE HEALTH AND MEDICAL ANTHROPOLOGY

Women's reproductive health is a complex domain involving effects that are both direct and indirect biological and social. Understanding the range of meaning of reproductive behaviours and beliefs within particular social and cultural settings, represent an important avenue for research in medical anthropology. Because of its long empirical tradition as well as its qualitative research strategy in ethnography, the discipline of anthropology and particularly the sub-discipline of medical anthropology represents a prime field for discovery of local reproductive norms and practices, including how individual living within communities define and experience their reproductive health and health problems. This focus on meaning and the lived experience of reproductive health, within particular local, cultural context, allows medical anthropologist to inform reproductive health discussion based on finding from epidemiology, demography and other sectors of international health, including population policy and family planning. The cultural meaning of reproduction will have a significant impact in understanding their own reproductive health status and this will influence in their health care seeking behaviour.

Medical anthropology has hitherto been conceived of as a tool for investigating and explicating local perspectives on reproductive health. Medical anthropological research often takes over where standard epidemiological and demographic research "leaves off by attempting to understand why women behave the way they do in the realm of reproductive relations." (Nations, M.K., 1986) Different societies encounter, define and experience different reproductive health problems biologically as well as culturally. A medical anthropological perspective emphasizes the diversity in local health needs and the importance of understanding that diversity in order to develop appropriate interventions. Medical anthropology has tended to describe cultural variation in health belief systems, emphasizing people's own descriptions and experience of reproductive health and illnesses within local cultural systems. It also examines how structures of inequality within and between the social groups cause, perpetuate and augment reproductive health problems.

1.5 EVOLUTION FROM BIRTH CONTROL TO REPRODUCTIVE HEALTH

Society has traversed a long way from the motivation to reduce population growth at any cost to a position in which individual rights and needs hold central stage. The focus on women's reproductive function, if not on women themselves, began and rapidly escalated in the 1960's with an urgent call for slower population growth. Between 1930's and 1960's the world had grown from 2 to 3 billion people, but by 1975 it had reached 4 billion. "Population control" acquired a pejorative reputation, however and hence "family planning" became the watchword of the 1970's.

However, the past decade witnessed emergence of an increased interest in women's reproductive health and development related programmes to improve reproductive health across the globe. This phenomenon was primarily catalyzed by the 1994 International conference on Population and Development (ICPD) in Cairo. The Cairo conference was the watershed that brought reproductive health into the international arena of population debates. This conference solidified a new, comprehensive understanding of reproductive health, largely owing to the effort of participating policymakers, researchers, health service providers, scholars, feminists and health advocates from developed and developing countries. ICPD was a radical departure from population rhetoric, a paradigm shift from a macro level focus to a micro level concern with individual rights in relation to sexuality and reproduction gaining ascendance over the demographic arguments for population policy. In September 1994 at the ICPD, 184-country government "reached an unprecedented consensus on a 20 year programme of action to achieve between the world's people and its resource. For the first time the reproductive and sexual health and reproductive rights of women became central to an international agreement on population (Germain, 1995).

1.5.1 Indian Scenario:

During much of the last 30 years, the Family Welfare Programme of the Ministry of Health and Family Welfare vigorously pursued a target approach to enhance contraceptive prevalence and to achieve the countries demographic goal of population stabilization. Family Planning has always persisted in India, driven by global hysteria about a possible population "explosion". "Target" oriented goals were met by holding sterilization camps reaching an extreme of forced sterilization in the mid 70's which led to the downfall of the then ruling political regime (Gandhi and Shah, 1993).

Concomitant to shift in women's health policy at a global level, a policy shift gradually appeared in India too. In 1995, the Ministry of Health and Welfare announce the removal of sterilization targets from Family Planning Programmes in 50 districts of India. Method specific targets were wiped out nationwide in April 1996. Though vociferous in their articulation and predicted chaotic outcomes for India (Ross, 1998) the population control policy, which was wedded to a top-down bureaucratic, having target driven system, came to an end after four decades of reign. Finally the government of India endorsed the new Programme of Action and in 1997 envisaged its translation into reality by introducing a reproductive and child health approach into its exiting Family Welfare Programme.

In order to broaden women's choices in all aspects of reproduction, the Fourth World Conference for Women in Beijing (UN, 1995) strongly advocated an empowerment approach. The approach involves empowering of women to have control over their own fertility and sexuality under condition of voluntary choice and minimum health risks. Several related factors precipitated this paradigm shift to reproductive health including -

1. An emphasis on reproductive and sexual rights by feminists in developing and developed countries (Correa and Reichmann, 1994; Petchesky, 2000).
2. The denunciation of population control as a motivation for

contraceptive research and distribution (Bandarage, 1997; Dixon-Mueller, 1993).

3. The need to address the HIV/AIDS pandemic and the increasing incidence of heterosexual transmission (Gates and Stone, 1992; Dixon- Mueller, 1993; Mbizuo, 1996; Parker, Barbosa and Aggleton, 2000).
4. The failure of family planning and maternal child health programmes to address complex reproductive health issues such as sexuality (Cliquet and Thienpont, 1995).

Thus in the post Cairo era, reproductive health has emerged as an organizational framework linking more traditional reproductive issues such as family planning and maternal and child health, with a suite of additional concerns, including STI (Sexually Transmitted Infections). The inclusion of reproductive health brings in reproductive tract infections including HIV/AIDS as a part of reproductive health concern. Women's reproductive health agenda thus embraces a wide array of concerns centered on reducing morbidity and mortality of women. It was spelled out and an eclectic agenda has heralded as a contentious but urgent issue goaded on one hand by the serious health problems faced by women and by concern about population growth, poverty and environmental degradation on other hand.

1.6 WOMEN'S REPRODUCTIVE HEALTH RESEARCH

The results of a number of community based prevalence studies of gynecological morbidity undertaken in the last decade, both in India (Koenig et al., 1998) and in other developing countries such as Nigeria, Turkey, Bangladesh and Egypt Brabin et al., 1995; Bulut et al., 1995; Wasserheit et al., 1989; Younis et al., 1993) have had to an increased awarness among researchers and policy makers, of the magnitude of RTI and their grave consequences among poor women. In India, these have been instrumental in placing the neglected issues of RTIs on the national policy agenda (Measham and Heaven, 1996).

1.6.1 Panoramic Review of Reproductive Health Research in Global Scene:

Beginning in the early 1990's, a series of inter-disciplinary community based studies has been carried out. Most of the researches on prevalence of reproductive morbidity in 1990's have focused on self-reported morbidity or women's perception of their health problem. In some studies, the women's self report were complemented with clinical and laboratory data and the degree of co-relation between women's perception of morbidity and medical definition of pathology were examined (Koenig et al., 1998). While a single community study cannot claim to be representation, it can identify reproductive health and associated morbidity as embedded in the local setting and related to issues such as women's understanding of their bodies, their access to health care and the gendered structure of domestic power. In Nigeria, participatory community based studies of reproductive health has involved community members in identifying the reproduction health problems and helping to solve them (Bang and Bang, 1996). Precedents for community study of reproductive health were reported in Egypt. The 10 years interdisciplinary study on the reproductive health study in Giza, on the urban fringe of Cairo, focused on 500 women in 2 villages.

Within Egypt, a number of ethnographic studies of rural women's health and status have provided insights into reproductive health although they did not focus on this topic *per se*. Younis et al. (1993) took up his study in rural Egypt with a sample size of 509 women. The study revealed that 52.0 percent of women had at least one reproductive tract infections, 56 percent had genital prolapse and 11 percent had abnormal cervical cell change. Similar study taken up by Maha Talaat et al. (2004) in Giza, Egypt revealed that 40 percent of women suffered from prolapse. Laboratory investigation showed an extremely high prevalence of chronic cervicitis (74.6 percent). Syphilis was detected in 11 women i.e. 13 percent and 9 percent of pelvic inflammation.

In a study conducted in rural area of Bangladesh, 2 percent of women were infected with chlamydia, 35 percent had bacterial vaginosis, 0.4 percent was positive for gonorrhea and 5 percent for trichomoniasis (Wasserheit, 1989). Overall, 68 percent of women were found to be suffering from one reproductive tract infection or the other.

In another study conducted in a Somali village (Ismail, 1990) syphilis was found in 2.25 percent of women and chlamydia infection was found in 18 percent of females.

Mosa's (1993) study in Tanzania revealed from serological evidence that syphilis was observed in 15.8 percent of women and reported 4.2 percent of genital ulcer. The corresponding proportions for urethral discharge or abnormal vaginal discharge were 28.0 percent and 7.1 percent respectively.

Zurayak.H. et al. (1995) conducted a study amongst 509 ever married non-pregnant women residing in two villages in Giza, (Egypt) and observed that 22 percent had bacterial vaginosis, 18 percent tichomoniasis, 11 percent candidiasis, 10 percent cervicitis and 2 percent of pelvic inflammatory disease.

Brabin, Kemb and Obunge (1995) conducted a study among adolescent girls in rural Nigeria to determine the prevalence of reproductive tract infections. They found that in their study sample of unmarried adolescents Nigerian girls, 42.1 percent had a reproductive tract infection.

A study was conducted at Istanbul (Turkey) among women aged between 15-44 years residing in the catchments area of maternal and child health at family planning clinic. The finding shows that 4.8 percent had bacterial vaginosis, 2.9 percent had cervicitis and 3.7 percent had pelvic inflammatory disease (Bulut, A., 1995).

The panoramic overview of reproductive health of women at the global domain shows heavy load of reproductive tract infection. Research work done in Egypt, Nigeria, Istanbul, Somali, Bangladesh shows heavy reproductive tract infection which calls for an urgency to address the problem.

1.6.2 Reproductive Health Research in India:

In Indian, context, some studies have brought to limelight the considerable brunt of reproductive morbidity among women. However, there is paucity of data due to female subservience in sexual and social matters and where taboo and silence limits the possibility of opening spaces for people to be able to express themselves and share their experiences. The reproductive health needs are culture specific and pose implicit difficulties in their understanding because of inherent inhibition, stigma and shame in the Indian context.

In India the 'wake up call" for research on women's reproductive health in India actually began before Cairo, with the landmark study by Bang and Bang (1989) form rural Maharastra. In this landmark study among rural tribal women, Bang and Bang (1989) demonstrates a high prevalence (92 percent) of reproductive morbidity in a sample of 650 women. There is a high prevalence of vaginal infection such as vaginalis (13.95 percent) candidiasis (34.5 percent) and syphilis (10.5 percent) (Bang, 1994). In the early part of the 1990's the Ford Foundation and other NGO's groups sponsored studies with a focus on women's perception of their health problem using qualitative methods. In some studies, the women's self report were complemented with clinical and laboratory data and the degree of correlalation between the women's perception of morbidity and medical definition of pathology was examined (Garg et al., 2000; Bhatia et al., 1997; Latha et al., 1997). Several other researchers have moved beyond parlance and explored women's perception of reproductive health problems. These studies have also explored the cognitive domains of illness and the ways in which women conceptualized these health problems (Bang and Bang, 1994).These studies have provided an understanding of reproductive morbidity in terms of etiology, symptoms and to some degree the severity of illness and health care seeking behaviour (Oomman, 1996).

The study of rural women in Karnataka by Bhatia and Cleland (1995) highlighted that 1/10 of the women had sexually transmitted diseases comprising of 7.5 percent trichomoniasis vaginalis, 0.8 percent gonorrhea, 1.5 percent of syphilis and 5.2 percent of candidiasis. A survey of 370 female sex workers in West Bengal revealed that 13.2 percent of these women were suffering from gonorrhea, 58.8 percent from syphilis, 11.1 percent from trichomoniasis and 23.2 percent from candidiasis (Singh, 1995).

Oomman (1996) conducted study in a Rajasthan village and has correlated vaginal discharge as a symptom with gynaecologist's examination and laboratory investigation. 194 women were reported having discharge and 131 were identified by the gynaecologist. The self reported symptom of discharge was also compared with the gynaecologist's diagnosis of either vaginitis/cervicitis. There was moderate accordance between women's self reported symptom and gynaecologist diagnosis. Comparison of laboratory investigation with the self reported symptom showed poor agreement.

These findings unraveled a heavy burden caused by reproductive morbidity among adolescent and women of the developing world. These reproductive illnesses among women are invisible because of the "culture of silence" that surrounds them and their inaccessibility to health care for these illnesses. Women have been bearing this burnt since time immemorial. Now, the time has come to create the space for voicing out the woes and agonies to attain their legitimate right and control over their body. There is a need to break down this silence.

1.7 REPRODUCTIVE TRACT INFECTION-A CAUSE OF CONCERN

In India and in other countries, the problem of reproductive tract infection is on the rise and these problem needs to be addressed and curtailed if a woman has to be given back her reproductive rights and responsibility. The management and control of reproductive tract infections, including the sexually transmitted infections at the grassroots level, is one of the paraphernalia of the reproductive health approach. In India, reproductive tract infections are very common. Studies have shown that 92 percent of women in the reproductive age suffer from different types of infections of reproductive tract (Bang and Bang, 1992). In Bangladesh 68 percent of women were found to be suffering from one reproductive tract infection or other (Wasserheit, 1989). Zurayak (1995) observed that 53 percent of women suffering from reproductive tract infections and 42.1 percent of unmarried adolescent Nigerian girls had reproductive tract infections (Brabin et al., 1995).

These findings indicate that there is a necessity for efficacious intervention to bring it under control. Reproductive tract infections have been largely ignored because of widespread belief that they rarely result in severe morbidity/mortality contrary to the reality which has potentially devastatingly sequeale.

There is a need to explore these areas in order to improve women's health. Oomman (1997) described women's report of reproducing morbidity in terms of their views about their body anatomy and physiology and the practices they follow in accordance with these beliefs. She also express the need to relate locally reported symptoms to western biomedical definition of disease especially in finding high prevalence of reproductive tract infections and that women are treated for infections on the basis of reported symptoms.

Health service provider must understand how women perceive the different types of RTI's and how they differ from biomedical categories of disease(Germain, 1992). At the same time, importance must be given to determine the risk factors of reproductive morbidity which affect women in developing countries. Although the biological risk factors may be universal, the cultural, social meaning of the illness will vary from one society to another. The risk factors that affect rural Egyptian women may or may not differentially affect rural Nigerian women. This knowledge will assist in providing a broad framework to health care provider in designing an efficacious, appropriate and sustainable and preventive intervention for reproductive health of women.

1.7.1 Sexually Transmitted Infection and HIV/AIDS:

The relationship between reproductive tract infections, sexually transmitted infections and HIV/AIDS is three-fold. Firstly, reproductive tract infections, sexually transmitted infections and HIV infection are associated with the same risk behaviour that is unprotected sexual intercourse with multiple partners.

Secondly, the presence of reproductive tract infections, sexually transmitted infections has been found to facilitate the acquisition and transmission of HIV infection. A ten-fold increased risk for HIV transmission has been associated with infections that cause genital ulcers, such as syphillis, chancroid, and herpes. The risk associated with diseases causing discharge, especially gonorrhea, chlamydial infection, trichomoniasis and bacterial vaginosis, is up to four-fold. Lastly, there is mounting evidence that some reproductive tract infection pathogens are more virulent in the presence of HIV related immune-deficiency (Mueller and Wasserheit, 1991).

Current evidence also strongly supports the facilitative role of sexually transmitted infections in spreading HIV/AIDS and drives home this point. Sexually transmitted genital ulcerative diseases - chancroid, syphilis, herpes and HIV-1 transmission (Finger, 1992) The recent result of a study carried out in Zaire also suggest trichomoniasis to be a risk factor for HIV-1 transmission (Laga et al., 1992).

The relationship between non ulcerative STI's such as gonorrhea, chlamydia and trichomoniasis, and HIV-1, has yet to be assessed. Nonetheless, as about 80 percent of HIV-1 infection is spread by sexual route, experts agree that in order to prevent the spread of HIV-1, a global initiative would be required in the prevention and control of STI's at the primary health care level (Adler, 1996).

India has had a national programme for the prevention and control of STI's since the 1960's but the services are either of poor quality, inaccessible, or socially unacceptable (Luthra et al, 1992; Nag, 1993; Ramasubban, 1996).

1.7.2 HIV/ AIDS Situation among Women:

Within the paradigm of reproductive health, another threatening and cause of serious concern is the pandemic rise of HIV/AIDS. Out of 40.3 million people living in this world with HIV/AIDS by December 2005, 17.5 million were women.

HIV is prevalent in almost all parts of the country. HIV/AIDS is spreading from urban to rural areas. HIV/AIDS is also spreading from high risk behaviour group to the general population, since early 1990. One in every four cases reported is a woman. About 89 percent of the reported cases are from the sexually active and economically productive age group of 15 - 49 years (NACO, 1998). In India 27 million women become pregnant every year of which 100,000 will be HIV positive. India has 1,029 billion populations and there are 4.58 million which is HIV infected by the end of December 2002. By the end of 2003, NACO has reported 57,781 AIDS cases in India which is grossly under reported because majority of the people with HIV/AIDS does not come to Government hospital for treatment. By the end of May 2005, the total number of HIV/AIDS cases reported in India was 109,399 of whom 31,982 were women (AIDS India, 2006).

Coming down to Manipur, till June 2004, the Manipur State Aids Control Society reported a seropositivity rate of 18.90 per 1000 and a total of 13,095 AIDS cases of which 2,066 were females (MACS, 2004).

1.8 ADDRESSING REPRODUCTIVE HEALTH NEEDS OF WOMEN IN INDIA

Reproductive health care is defined as a constellation of methods, techniques and services that contribute to reproductive health and well being by preventing and solving reproductive health problem. Significant progress has been made over the past few decades in providing health care to people in India. But this progress has not been egalitarian, as women; in particular have not had an equal share. The elements required for woman to have effective access to care are myriad and complex. While ensuring the availability of facilities and personnel within reasonable distance is indeed a primary requirement, effective access to care can only be ensured if that care is considered affordable, appropriate and acceptable by the women it aims to serve. Women in India face constraints, not only in obtaining services, but also in expressing their reproductive health needs (Gittelsohn et al., 1994). Lack of awareness, cultural barriers and economic factors prevent them from seeking timely care. Research in India shows that poor women carry a heavy burden of reproductive morbidity; a significant component of such morbidity is unrelated to pregnancy and is due to reproductive tract infections, many of which are sexually transmitted; the reproductive illnesses among women are invisible because of the "culture of silence" that surrounds them; and women do not have access to health care for these illnesses. As past programmes have recognized women only as mothers, many women were not served and many reproductive health problems not addressed. (Pachauri, 1994). Moreover, women only seek for assistance when condition become severe and secondary complication arises.

Women are relatively unlikely to seek advice when there is a tendency to view morbidities such as white discharge as normal and when the condition is often associated with shame or guilt, owing to its perceived link with promiscuity. Further, most women with a lower reproductive tract infections are asymptomatic. Pelvic examination is strongly resisted by all women, but more so if they are asymptomatic and especially, if they are to be performed by health service providers who are not sensitive to their needs. With restriction in women's mobility and lack of autonomy in decision making it is unlikely that they will take the initiative in obtaining health care for themselves.

In India a variety of health care systems co-exist namely: Allopathy, Ayurveda, Sidhha, Unani, Nature Cure and Yoga (Baltiwala, 1988). People access different systems for different illnesses or even for the same illness episode, a phenomenon which is found in many western and non-western societies (Helman, 1990).

1.8.1 Health Care System in Rural India:

The health services available to women in rural India comprises of government health services, traditional care including home remedies. The government provides health services to the rural poor through a network of Primary Health Centres (PHCs), sub-centres and referral centres called Community Health Centre (CHC's). A sub-centre provides services to a population of 5000 while there is one PHC for every 30,000 population and one CHC for every 100,000 to 120,000 population. The government also places Auxiliary Nurse Midwives (ANM) to work with Traditional Birth Attendants (TBA's) at the village level. In cities and towns, the government provides health services through a network of government and municipal hospitals, dispensaries and family welfare centres (IIPS, 1995).

For a women living in a village factors such as distance from the site of care, lack of availability of equipment and supplies at the site and lack of money to cover the cost of transportation and treatment are the key constraints to access care. Lack of time and money as well as availability of health facilities play important role in delaying health care seeking by women (Bang and Bang, 1994; Narayan and Srinivasan, 1994). Women overcome their limitation by using home remedies and consulting traditional healers who are mostly men (Gandhi and Shah 1993) for their physical, social and psychological problems. Traditional birth attendants, the only female healers in a village, are generally consulted for health problems related to pregnancy and child birth and gynecological problems. When homes remedies do not work, women in rural India resort to "private" practitioners who have little or no allopathic training and treat women according to the system of Ayurveda and Unani (Jeffery et al., 1989). In corollary, there are number of quack doctors who are not trained in Allopathy but prescribe an admixture of allopathic and ayurvedic medicine to patients. As Nichter (1989) reports, there is co-modification of health occurring in India causing people to loose their traditional knowledge of home remedies as they increasingly came in contact with western medicine.

There is paucity of data regarding access of health care system by women in India. As long as the ailment does not disturb their daily chores it is visualized as "a part of life" and women frequently resort to self medication. The existing socio-cultural barriers and taboos associated with diseases even remotely connected with reproduction and sexuality are major hindrances to women seeking help for reproductive tract infections (Luthra et al., 1991). Women initially ignore their symptoms but seek treatment only when their symptoms increase in severity (Kanani, Latha and Shah, 1994).

1.8.2 Potent Obstacle:

Distance limits women's willingness and ability to seek care, particularly when appropriate transportation is in limited supply, communications difficult, and terrain and climate inhospitable. In India's Ananthapur District, women transported to the hospital with serious pregnancy related complication, 69 percent went by public bus and 19 percent by animal drawn carts (Bhatia 1986 as cited in Thaddeus and Maine 1990).

1.8.3 Access to Care: More than a Problem of Distance in India:

Women often feel that government health centers are deficient in several ways: they are not open at convenient hours for women. Often they are located far away from some villages, although health centres are supposed to provide free services, villagers are often charged for services and one is required to buy medical supplies from market, staff are rude to villagers and treat them with little respect; government doctors are usually male, making it difficult for a women to approach them especially for gynecological problem (Jeffery et al., 1989) Traditional remedies are often the first line of health care sought, including some remedies that may introduce or exacerbate infection (Kanani et at., 1994).

Thus, the health care systems of rural India might be characterized by a different set of "four too's": too far from home, too few trained birth attendants, too poorly equipped to identity or handle complication and too deficient in quality of care.

1.9 SELECTION OF SITE AND TOPIC

Ratiocinating from the following points, I have conducted my study in Manipur-

(1) Reproductive health of women in Manipur has hitherto been an unexplored area.

(2) Manipur is a poverty stricken state with poor infrastructure and poor utilization of health care services by the people for RTI's.

(3) HIV/AIDS is pandemic in Manipur.

The preliminary research findings indicating high level of reported symptoms of reproductive tract infection enthused me to work in this area of study. Findings from Egypt, India, and Nigeria direct towards this point. This study will endeavour to find out the magnitude of RTI's and identify its cultural, environmental and social correlates. It seek to answer my inquisitive mind regarding the women's perception of reproductive morbidity in term of biology, progression and symptoms of illness, whether it goes in congruence with a clinically diagnosed morbidity or it measures a different phenomenon. This study will endeavour to explore women's perception of their body parts–how the different body parts function i.e. the ethno-gynaecology of Andro which will help in shaping out the etiology, progression of reproductive ailments.

The study scrutinizes the factors influencing the risk of RTI's including personal social, cultural, demographic, obstetric and reproduction history use of contraception, hygiene, behaviour and health care seeking behaviour. Epidemiological tools have been employed to explore the differences in reproductive morbidity (self reported), different patterns of seeking health care between the two communities.

Last but not the least this study also focuses on the impact of government policies and programmes on reproductive health needs of the women in Manipur, the difficulties and problem faced by the women in accessing the health.

1.10 OBJECTIVE OF THE STUDY

The main objectives of this study are given below:

1. To study the magnitude of RTI's.
2. To explore women's perception of body, reproductive illnesses and health seeking behavior.
3. To compare women's reported symptom with clinical examination and laboratory test results.
4. Assess factors influencing the risks of RTI's including personal, social, cultural, demographic, obstetric, reproductive history, use of contraception and hygiene.
5. Compare between Andro and Kwakeithel:

a. Differences in reproductive health morbidity

b. Differences in health seeking patterns

c. Risk factors of RTI's

6. To provide a basis for recommendation to health and family planning programmes.

Thus, this chapter discusses on how reproductive caliber of women is complemented with hazardous health consequences which are inflicted from sex, pregnancy, childbirth, abortion and improper use of contraceptive methods posing a threat to the reproductive health of women worldwide. It also discusses on why incorporation of epidemiology is essential in the reproductive health studies. Because of its long empirical tradition as well as its qualitative research strategy, medical anthropology represents a prime field for discovery of local reproduction norms and practices including how individual living within the communities define and experience their reproductive health and reproductive health problems. This chapter also discusses on the paradigm shift in government policy and programmes from population rhetoric to individual rights in relation to sexuality and reproduction and the heavy burden of reproductive tract infection as evidenced from the research work reported both in the International domain as well as in the Indian context which needs to be addressed.

2

Theoretical Framework and Literature Review

2.1 THE MEANING OF HEALTH

The meaning of health is culturally defined. Therefore understanding of the women's perception of reproductive health is a sine qua non in order to give a pictographical (holistic) representation of women's health. The concept of perceived morbidity has been included in the framework of this study and therefore there is a need to understand the conceptual distinctions between "disease" and "illness" which was firstly augmented in the seventies by psychiatrist/medical anthropologists (Kleinman, Eisenberg and Good, 1978) medical anthropologist (Fabrega, 1972). The concept of disease has historically been the most dominant category; it has a biological interpretation and refers to abnormalities in the structure or function of organs and organ systems, pathological states whether or not they are culturally recognized. Health, as a felt experience of the individual, provides another meaning which is embodied in the term "illness". Thus, illness is the meaning that individual give to health and refers to a "person" disvalued states including but not limited to disease (Young, 1982). Illness is the individual's consciousness that there is something wrong. (Frankenberg, 1980).

2.1.1 Illness and Sickness:

Disease in the western medical paradigm is malfunctioning or maladaptation of biologic and psycho physiologic processes in the individual, whereas illness represents personal, interpersonal and cultural reactions to disease and/or discomfort. Illness is shaped by cultural factors governing perception, labeling explanation, and valuation of the discomforting experience, processes embedded in a complex family, social and cultural nexus. Because illness experience is an intimate part of social systems of meaning and rules for behaviour, it is strongly influenced by culture: it is, as we shall see, culturally constructed (Kleinman, Eisenberg and Good, 1978).

In dealing with the concept of perceived morbidity, the role of socio-cultural factors becomes apparent not only as a determinant of the occurrence of illness, but also as essential in the construction of the concept of ill-health. In fact, this important role of socio cultural factor goes beyond the individual to act on society's construction of health, through its determination of the break points marking degrees of good health and ill health on the health illness continuum representing health status (Johansson, 1991). As such these breakpoints are mostly "culturally negotiated". They are determined in order to ensure attention to problems considered serious in that culture.

This recognition of the role of socio-cultured factors in the production and distribution of health had led to another expression of meaning of health which is categorized as sickness (Frankenberg, 1980; Young, 1982). Sickness includes both disease and illness in being the process of the "making social of disease" (Frankenberg, 1980). In fact, neither disease nor illness are separate entities but rather explanatory models held by a provider versus a patient to explain the phenomenon of sickness. The dynamic interplay between biological, psychological and socio-cultural factors need to be understood for effective treatment of single phenomena adumbrated as "sickness".

Reproductive illness is not only a biological but is embedded in a web of psychological, economic, political and social factor. There is a gross lack of information on socio-cultural context: values, customs and social status, the socialization processes and the concept of sexuality were not adequately explored. Different societies encounter, define and experience different reproductive health problems biologically as well as culturally. Different cultures define reproductive illness in different context and what is recognized as reproductive illness may not be so in others. For this study, reproductive illness refers to illness which women perceive as related to their sexual and reproductive organs and functioning. On the other hand reproductive morbidity refers to diseases or condition of women's reproductive systems as defined from the biomedical standpoint. There is a need to unravel these dimensions to dig out the real facet of reproductive illness of women.

2.2 RETROSPECT OF WOMEN'S REPRODUCTIVE HEALTH RESEARCH

Medical anthropology has hitherto been conceived of as a tool for investigating and explicating local perspective on reproductive health. Medical anthropologist has always tended to describe cultural variation in health belief systems, emphasizing on people's own description and experience of reproductive health and illnesses within local cultural system. They make an endeavor to understand the people's perception of their bodies, the location of different parts of the body, the interrelationship of different parts of the body, their functions, etc. to give an account of "bodily basis of illnesses". Thus, to get the zest of the aspects of reproductive health of women it is necessary to elicit information as to what knowledge women have regarding their own body, reproductive organs and their functioning which is also known as ethno-anatomy and ethno- physiology.

Medical anthropologist ethnographic work focused on fertility and childbirth prior to the advent of feminist perspective in medical anthropology. Since then, researchers began to focus on women's perceptions of their own health.

2.2.1 Cultural Construction of Fertility and Child birth:

Pertinent to child bearing and fertility there is a plethora of work particularly topics relevant to women's perception on childbirth. Studies focusing on issues of birth attendants, labor management, childbirth pollution, food and mishaps in deliveries are also not less common. Mac Cormack (1982), edited a collection of essays on the cultural construction of fertility and birth in countries ranging from Sri Lanka, New Guinea, Sierra Leone, and Ghana to Britain to demonstrate the wide range of cultural rules and social practices that exist in all societies and influence fertility and child birth. In India, Jeffery et al.(1981) laments out the women's voices reflecting on their experiences of child bearing and provided an accessible and existing reassessment of women's roles in an agricultural society traversing a women's life from the time they marry via the moment they enter their husband's household till they give birth. Nichter (1989), in his South Asian case studies examined the cultural notions of fertility in Sri Lanka and its impact on family planning practices. He also wrote about findings on ethno-physiology and food consumption practices during pregnancy in South India. Nichter (1981), demonstrated that South Indian women eat less during pregnancy so that they will deliver small babies, not just to ease the birth process but rather to give their bodies more space inside their womb while they are growing. Women in this study reported that if they ate a lot during pregnancy, the food would occupy the "baby space" inside them preventing a baby from growing (Nichter, 1981).

Corollary to such ethnographic work, public health initiatives such as safe motherhood has also included women's perceptions of childbirth in programme to improve maternal and neonatal health (SEWA Rural, 1994). Another conceptualization is the parental care. To drive home this point is the work done by Adetunji (1996). He describes the traditional conceptualization of parental care in a Nigerian community and draws its implication for effective delivery of reproductive health services in the area. The findings highlights a local metaphor that linked the risks of pregnancy and childbirth to a group of women that trekked to a local brook to fetch water with their earthen pots, some fell, broke their pots, some missed steps and spilt their water but kept their pots and others returned without any mishap. The first group represented cases of maternal mortality, the second groups were cases of miscarriage, stillbirths or infants death, and the third group represented successful outcome for both pregnancy and the resultant baby. From the findings few conclusion emerge such as the existing concept of parental care and reproductive health in this community. The reproductive health described conceptualized both maternal and child health care as inseparable and that maternal health is inherently important for child health. The traditional prenatal care included the idea of physical as well as metaphysical sources of illness and tried to combat both, whereas the modern care focuses only on the physical.

2.2.2 Women's Perception of Reproductive Health and Patterns of Health Care in the Global Scenario:

Many studies were carried out to understand people's perception of different illnesses or bodily composition. Young (1981), in his study of the community of Pichataro in Mexico, attempted to understand illnesses which people mentioned in terms of their perceptions of their bodies. On the basis of his findings, he showed how men and women made "medical choices" to treat their illnesses and how these choices varied according to the beliefs about the causes of illnesses.

Within Egypt, a number of ethnographic/anthropological studies of rural women's health and status have provided insights into reproductive health. Maha Talaat et al., (2004) conducted a year long interdisciplinary study to identify female genital schistosomiasis in an Egyptian hamlet. Clinical assessment was combined with an in-depth study of the social context of reproductive health. Along with 16.7 percent of women having *Schistosomia haebatobuim* other reproductive tract morbidities were also identified. Clinical examination revealed that 39.5 percent of women suffered from viginitis and more than half i.e. 53.3 percent from prolapse. Laboratory investigations showed an extremely high prevalence of chronic cervicitis, 75.6 percent syphilis was detected in 13.1 percent of women. The study identified a number of factors that would affect the reproductive health care in general. General neglect of women's health especially relating to reproductive health was one of the general concerns.

It was found that women were unwilling to complain to their husband if they are unwell for fear that they will take another wife or divorce them nor do they discuss these problems with female kins and friends for fear of stigmatization and shame. Another profound finding is the prevailing fatalism about health problem, the belief that many are normal or conditions that cannot be treated, is also associated with women's limited awareness of their bodies and their reproductive system. Many women regarded uterine prolapse as "normal" so long as it does not interfere with delivery or intercourse. Women knew little about prolapse. Some of them had been told about it by the *daya* (traditional birth attendant) during delivery, as she attempted to push it back by hand. A few women identified it and linked it to the protrusion of an egg like mass, the local term for prolapse is *beit elweld saket* literally, "when the uterus comes down like on egg". Discharge was referred to variously as *rhima, marawed, raghaury* and *seila*. Another finding from this study is misconceptions about family planning and revelation of limited access and use of health care. There is no health center or private doctor in this hamlet and no regular transport to the nearest Rural Health Unit, which is 3 km away. Although there are a number of traditional health care system providers, none of them address the reproductive health problem *per se,* although they address the problem of infertility. There are two *dayas* (traditional birth attendants), who oversee all the deliveries in the hamlet. One of them, who was over 90 years , recruited to attend the delivery as it was considered to have *baraka,* which brings good fortune to the family.

Pimpawun Boonmongkon et al., (2001), documented from North East Thailand women's experiences of gynecological complaint which broadly encompass symptoms commonly associated with RTI's and pelvic, lower abdominal and back pain associated with hard manual labor, childbearing, menstruation, etc as well as other symptoms linked to the "uterus" (*mot luuk*) through cultural reasoning. Boonmongkon et al. examined the women's explanatory models about what ailed them, levels of concern associated with persistent complaints, forms of self treatment, and pattern of health care seeking, as well as the types and quality of health services available to women. This was an intensive focused ethnographic study that aimed at achieving a more in-depth understanding of ethno-gynaecology, women's interpretations of symptoms and the progression of illness, physical and psychological suffering and health seeking strategies. In North East Thailand, women suffer from *mot luuk* problems, regardless of whether or not they have a disease that doctors classify as significant and worthy of treatment. Women's experiences of *mot luuk* problems are influenced by a complex of factors, including the burden of women's work, perceptions of illness causality that carry social significance, fears that sexual relations will aggravate symptoms and lead to cervical cancer, additional fears that they will lose their husbands to other women if sexual relations are suspended.

Seven explanatory model of illness causality by women suffering from chronic or recurrent *mot luuk* problems were developed by Boonmongkon (2001).

(1) Ulcer model: An ulcer inside the *mot luuk* gets infected and full of pus, fungus/germs make the ulcer worse, discharge often occurs and the woman gets cancer.

(2) Husband infects wife model: The husband has extramarital sex

with a woman who is not clean and transfers fungus or germs to his wife who gets a *mot luuk* problem, discharge with bad odor occurs and sometimes itching. The woman develops *mot luuk ak seep* (inflammation/infection of the uterus) and an ulcer and gets cancer.

(3) Poor hygiene model: The *mot luuk* becomes infected from a woman working in a dirty place, dirt entering her body from a rice field or fish pond, not being able to wash after urination while working or dirt transferred to her sexually from a man with poor hygiene. Fungus/germs cause itching and bad odour and discharge occurs leading to cancer.

(4) Hard work model:Hard work leads to lower abdominal pain; the woman gets *jep mot luuk* (pain in the uterus) and/or *mot luuk ak seep* (inflammation/infection of the uterus) which can become cancer.

(5) IUD model:An IUD left inside for a long time causes an ulcer which becomes infected; discharge increases and woman gets cancer. *Yun fai* model: After delivery of a child, a woman does not stay by the fire to dry out her *mot luuk*; discharge increases, fungus/germs develop and she can get cancer.

(6) Sterilization model: Sterilization causes a woman to develop *mot luuk boo dii* (a bad uterus) which leads to cancer.

This study also documents the dangers of women's self treatment practices that rely largely on small doses of medically inappropriate antibiotics. Fungal infections are exacerbated by the use of antibiotics. Popular brands of tetracycline are widely believed to be 'good for *mot luuk* problems' in general and also capable of improving the condition of bad uterus (Boonmongbon et al., 2001).

The idea of taking tetracycline for *mot luuk* problems is not merely a 'folk medical belief' for these medicines are marketed through poster and radio advertising as drugs to treat the uterus (Boonmongkon, Nichter, Pylypa and Chantapasa, 1998; Whittaker, 1996). This study thus, provides details of women's perception about cause, effects and treatment of reproductive illness.

Another study by Lubma Ishaq Bhatti et al. (2002), explores the contextual factors influencing health seeking behaviour of women in Karachi regarding RTI. Causes of RTI reported were "melting bones" consuming food with perceived hot composition, poor personal hygiene and procedures like dilatation and curettage, delivery and induced abortion. Interference with religious activities, sexual relationship or socializing was reported as a consequence of RTI in addition to lower abdominal pain, menstrual irregularities, backache and weakness.

Alfamia Kaddour et al. (2005), elicit the definition of the concept of reproductive health among women in three communities around Beirut, Lebanon. The women's understanding of good reproductive health included three major themes, which were expressed differently in the three communities. Their understanding included good physical and mental health, their ability to reproduce and raise children, practice family planning and birth spacing, and going through pregnancy and motherhood safely were central to their reproductive duties, and their social status. Finally, they saw reproductive health within the context of economic status, good marital relations and strength to cope with their lives.

2.2.3 An Overview of Reproductive Health Research in Indian Context:

Few countable works have been done in India about women's perceptions of their reproductive health. One remarkable exception to this is Nichter's work in South India (Nichter 1981). On examining the idioms of distress, Nichter demonstrated a variety of alternative terms used by women to express psychological distress. Havik women of South India were found to express distress using cultural modes or idioms which Nichter categories as (1) food, weight loss, fasting and poisoning (2) purity (3) illness (4) spirits and evil eye and (5) devotion. The example which can be cited is expression of distress or conflict by a woman in terms of giving up certain foods or fasting completely or going on a pilgrimage to leave a stressful situation behind and seeking blessings from God.

In his study, another interesting aspect concerning women's illnesses is the illness idiom. Of a hundred women who visited a traditional ayurvedic healer 39percent complained of leucorrhoea (Nichter's term) 2.7 percent had menstrual complaints and 66 percent complained of weakness/ bloodlessness among other complaints of headaches, dizziness, body aches and disturbed sleep. Women believed that *bili hoguvudu* (white going) was due to dissolving bones or due to *dhatu* loss. *Dhatu* is considered an essential body humor that is associated with vitality, regulation of body processes, heat regulation, capacity to endure strength and a source of health. Semen is considered as *dhatu* which is a reservoir of both men and women (Obeyesekere, 1976). Nichter found that most of the 39 women who presented themselves with *bili hoguvudu* were suffering from some form of distress conflicts with other women in the family, sexual frustration or excessive sex or economic problem within the household. Therefore, women believed that they are suffering from *dhatu* loss and that their vitality and well being are slipping away.

In line with this, according to Nichter, women call for attention using menstrual complaints to direct attention to the "social, emotional and biological instability as well as impurity, social distance and marginality" they are subjected to during menstrual period. Subsequently, most women sought treatment for the above illnesses from a traditional healer and not a physician because they felt that a *vaidya* would restore "their health and well being" and not just treat their illness based on a set of physical symptoms (Nichter, 1981).

Many of those employing self-report methodology have focused attention on local illness terminology, and some have recognized the importance of studying the cultural meanings of the words such as "weakness" when used to describe gynecological problems (Bang and Bang, 1994).

Self reported data on reproductive morbidity has shown high reporting rates of *safed pani* (white water). The work done by Bang and Bang (1989) in rural Maharastra was an "eye opener". 95 percent of women were reported having vaginal discharge which were considered as the most serious and common health problem. Some evidence suggests that women may perceive white discharge as part of sexual maturation and consider it normal. The study also found that women had twelve terms for white discharge indicating that *safed pani* might be a term used to describe more than clinically defined discharge. Some exploration of this term was conducted to reveal perceived causes of *safed pani.* Women believe that they might get *safed pani* because their husbands have visited commercial sex workers. Some believe that contraception (tubectomy, IUD, oral pills, vasectomy) might cause white discharge, while others said that sexual dreams caused *kamjori* (weakness) which seems to be used concomitantly with *safed pani*. Other cause cited is witchcraft or black magic (Bang and Bang, 1992; 1994).

Women's perception of the effects of white discharge was also examined in the Bang and Bang study. Women with *safed pani* feel that they are losing their strength and therefore, use the terms *kamjori* (weakness) and *safed pani* (white discharge) interchangeably. Long terms effects of *safed pani* described by women include sterility and cancer (Bang and Bang, 1992; 1994). Although Bang and Bang (1989) were able to demonstrate high level of gynecological infection and conditions concomitant with frequent reports of discharge by women, they did not demonstrate the comparability (sensitivity, specificity, predictive values, agreement) of reported symptoms with presence of disease in their study. However, the qualitative phase of their study on women's perceptions of discharge does provide an insight into the many dimensions (physical, mental and sexual) of symptom in terms of discharge and weakness.

Several non-governmental organizations (NGO's) in India have taken up studies to understand women's reported symptoms of reproductive illnesses and epidemiology of reproductive morbidities. A number of studies on reproductive morbidities have been undertaken in India mainly in rural and urban areas of Gujarat (Patel, 1994; SEWA Rural Research team, 1994; Kanani et al., 1994; Patel et al., 1994), Maharashtra (Bang and Bang, 1994; Mulgaonkar et al., 1994; George, 1994), Tamil Nadu (Narayan et al., 1994), Karnataka (Bhatia and Cleland, 1995), Rajas than (Oomman, 1996), Kerela (Shenoy K.T. et al., 1997),

The main findings (Pachauri and Gittelsohn 1994) from the studies in India throw considerable light on Indian women's perceptions of their health. Vaginal discharge was the major complaint made by women. Twelve different terms were used for white discharge. "Weakness" is the perceived causal agent of white discharge or the perceived effect of discharge. The term "weakness" covers a wider connotation. It is used to vocalize any health problem. 'Weakness" is a generic term encompassing any and all symptoms of physical, mental and sexual discomfort and hence carried a wider meaning than is generally grasped by most allopathic health professionals. Most women felt that the common cause for white discharge was excessive heat bursting out from inside the body. Excessive heat may be caused by inherent body constitution. White discharge is also thought to be a disease of the uterus. Many believe that sore develop in the uterus, which burst open and the pus drains out in the form of white discharge. These women had their own perception of the causes of white discharge, perception far removed from reality.

In terms of severity, some women report discharge as the most severe illness, while in other areas women describe different forms of discharge, some more severe than the other. In these studies, women try to link discharge with other illnesses like weakness and backaches and use these as euphemisms to report discharge ratiocinating on the factors that attributed discharge as shameful. In some areas, discharge was associated with infidelity either on the part of the women or her husband. Additionally, women recognize clusters of symptoms which they report together because they experience them concurrently.

Based on a meta-analysis of eight studies in India, Pachauri and Gittelsohn (1994), constructed on ethno-medical model of women's illnesses. According to this model, Indian women attribute discharge, syphilis and menstrual problems to a variety of causes such as eating "hot" foods and having extramarital sex, witchcraft, physical work and tubectomy, sterilization operations. Once they have these illnesses women describe effects of these illnesses which include weakness, loss of productivity, anxiety, stress and cancer. Treatments sought for such illnesses vary from home remedies to traditional healer to allopathic healers depending on the location of the study. Home remedies were found to include different foods and herbs based on "hot-cold" classification of diseases i.e. women eat cooling foods to reduce the excess heat in their bodies that cause discharge. The response of women for not seeking treatment at gynecological health centers varied from lack of money and time to the lack of a sense of need of a gynecological examination. This study gives a pictographical presentation of women's perception of their reproductive illnesses. However, it lacked the clinical and laboratory examination as well as the comparison of women' perception of reproductive morbidity with the actual presence of gynecological condition.

Studies were also conducted based on women's report of gynecological illness without an investigation of women's perceptions of these illnesses.

Shatrugna et al. (1993), studied on the effect of women's work on their reproductive morbidity in a large urban slum showed that in a sample of ill women workers, almost 30 percent complains of gynecological morbidity, the highest category among all other complaints which included "general feelings of ill health," urinary problems, fevers and pregnancy and operation related problems. More women who worked for wages and women who are self employed reported gynecological complaints and general feelings of ill health compared to women who worked with their husband or families and women who are housewives.

The study by Bhatia and Cleland (1995), presents analysis of self-reported symptoms to examine the determinants of reproductive morbidity. Reported symptoms of abnormal discharge were assumed to correlate with lower reproductive tract (LRTI's) infection, reports of bleeding problem with menstrual problems, lower abdominal pain/discharge and fever with acute pelvic inflammatory disease (PID) and excessive weakness with anemia among other disease categories. Based on this categorization, 23.4 percent of women were found to have anemia, 16.9 percent had LRTI's, 7.3 percent had menstrual problems and 5.2 percent had acute PID. Other conditions reported by less than 2 percent of women included hemorrhoids, urinary infections, prolapse, fistulas and infertility. The study also found that significant predictors of the above four main outcomes were related to a woman's last pregnancy related problem, last place of delivery and whether a woman was sterilized or not. Additionally, the study suggested that in the light of general clinical practice in India symptoms may serve as a good indicator to refer women for further medical examinations. Though Bhatia and Cleland provides some significant findings in terms of addressing policy and treatment issues about women's health in India, one lacunae is its assumption that women's reported symptoms correlate with presence of biomedically defined disease/condition. Although the researchers mentioned that they do not consider reported symptoms to be diagnostically accurate, they carried out the determinant analysis based on this assumption. Thus, there is necessity to compare symptoms or complaints reported by women with medically diagnosed disorders/conditions. Furthermore, there is a lack of information on the sexual, behavioural and socio-cultural practices and beliefs of Indian women (Luthra et al., 1992).

Oomman (1996), in her study in a Rajasthan village emphasized on women's reproductive morbidity within its socio-economic and cultural context and was supplemented with clinical examination as well as laboratory test. This study demonstrated that rural Indian women have perceptions about their bodies and illnesses that are strongly related to the fact that they are "women", a term that embodies their low status due to poverty and gender inequality. Furthermore, women's perceptions of illness affect their actual health seeking behaviour as well as the way in which they will articulate a symptom or illness term to a health provider.

An ethno-medical model was developed on the basis of women's perception of severity of "women's illnesses" which include *dhola pani* (discharge), *kapda ro bimari* (menstrual problems) and *sharir bahar aave* (prolapse). The ethno-medical model suggests a similar mode of illness causation to a biomedical framework for determinants of morbidity. Based on a linear model, it appears that women see *ghar ki kamjori* (economic weakness/poverty) as the root cause of illness. Conditions directly resulting from poverty include anger, worry and anxiety, lack of food to eat and long days of work. These conditions produce *kamjori* (physiological weakness) which makes women susceptible to illnesses associated with sterilization operations, copper-T use, abortions, and delivery problems, eating hot foods, sexual intercourse and lifting heavy weights. Women have a sense of illness pathology, reflected in the above factors. The resulting common illnesses are *dhola pani* (white water) *kapda ro bimari* (menstrual problems) and *sharir bahar aave* (prolapse).

2.3 REPRODUCTIVE MORBIDITY

Reproductive morbidity (RM) is defined as 'any morbidity or dysfunction of the reproductive tract or any morbidity which is a consequence of reproductive behaviour including pregnancy, abortions, childbirths or sexual behaviour' (World Health Organization, 1996). According to Zurayk et al. (1993) and Oomman (2000), reproductive morbidity refers to conditions of ill health related to the reproductive process during and outside the childbearing period. Reproductive morbidity has been classified into three types: obstetric, gynecological and contraceptive (Zurayk et al., 1993). Obstetric morbidity can be defined as ill health related to pregnancy episode. Gynecological morbidity can be defined as structural and functional disorder of the reproductive tract not related to pregnancy, delivery and puerperum, basically diagnosed by clinical and laboratory tests. Contraceptive morbidity refers to morbidity caused by use of contraceptives. Obstetric morbidity will not be addressed in this dissertation. This study will focus primarily on gynecological morbidity including Reproductive Tract Infections (RTI's) in the light of the most frequently reported complaints by Indian women of vaginal discharge. Other gynaecologial problem like prolapse will also be included in this study.

2.3.1 Etiology and Definition of Reproductive Tract Infections:

Reproductive tract infections (RTI's) are being increasingly recognized as a serious global health problem. Female reproductive tract infections or RTI's is a generic term that covers three types of infection (Wasserheit, 1990). These infections may be bacterial, viral or protozoal infections of the lower and upper tract of males and females, although they affect men and women differentially (Wasserheit, 1992; Jacobson, 1991).

RTI's refer to three different types of infection:

(1) Endogenous infection is probably the most common RTI's worldwide. They result from an overgrowth of organisms normally present in the vagina. Endogenous infections include bacterial vaginosis and candidiasis. These infections can be easily treated and cured.

(2) Iatrogenic infections occur when the cause of infection (a bacterium or other micro organism) is introduced into the reproductive tract through a medical procedure such as menstrual regulation, induced abortion, insertion of an IUD or during childbirth. This can happen if surgical instruments used during the procedure have not been properly sterilized, or if an infection that was already present in the lower reproductive tract is pushed through the cervix into the upper reproductive tract.

(3) Sexually transmitted infections (STI's) are caused by viruses, bacteria or parasitic microorganisms that are transmitted through sexual activity with an infected partner. About 30 different sexually transmitted infections have been identified, some of

which are easily treatable, many of which are not. HIV, the virus that causes AIDS, is the most endangered sexually transmitted infection as it eventually leads to death.

All RTI are preventable. Moreover, all, except some of those caused by viruses are curable. But, the prevention, treatment and control of RTI's are unfortunately a complex and control of RTI's is unfortunately a complex issue. A multitude of factors-psychological, economic, political and social-faster their spread and must be addressed if RTI's are to be brought under control (Dixon-Mueller and Wasserheit, 1991).

(i) ***Diagnosis of Pelvic Inflammatory disease (PID):***

The definition and diagnosis of PID still remains to be a moot issue, preventing an accurate assessment of its etiology and prevalence in the developing and developed world (Jossens and Sweet, 1993). The difficulty in diagnosing. PID based on clinical findings lies in the fact that women present with a wide range of non-specific symptoms and sign. These symptom and sign vary from mild and vague symptoms to more accurate symptoms such as abnormal discharge and fever (CDC, 1991). According to CDC diagnosis can be difficult because the symptom may be subtle, vague or mild. There are no specific tests for PID so; diagnosis is usually based on a detailed health history, physical examination, blood test and sometimes various cultures. Pelvic ultrasound or other diagnostic procedures may be used. Although laparoscopic investigation of PID is considered the best diagnostic tool, it has been suggested that diagnostic errors can also occur with this procedure (Eschenbach, 1980) as well as complications that may be associated with any surgery (Dodson and Faro, 1985). Furthermore, laparoscopy is an economically and logistically impractical procedure for routine use in the developing and developed world. Consequently, PID is clinically diagnosed in most setting and sometimes supplemented with results from laboratory tests on including test on samples of vaginal discharge (CDC, 1991). To curb the problem in diagnosing the PID, CDC has made recommendation:

Minimum criteria for clinical diagnosis of PID:

1. Lower abdominal tenderness
2. Bilateral adnexal tenderness
3. Cervical motion tenderness

To increase the specificity of the diagnosis (i.e. to avoid false positives) the following criteria are added

Routine Additional Criteria:

1. Temperature greater than 38°C.
2. Abnormal cervical or vaginal discharge.
3. Elevated erythrocyte sedimentation rate or C-reactive protein.
4. Culture or non culture evidence of cervical infection with N. gonorrhea or C. trachomatis

Elaborate additional Criteria:

1. Histopathologic evidence on endiometrial biopsy.
2. Tubo ovarian abscess on sonography
3. Laparoscopy.

Bacteriological Test recommended for all suspected cases of PID:

1. Cervical cultures for N. gonorrhea
2. Cervical culture or non culture test for C. trachomatis.

of RTI:

Sequeale of RTI:

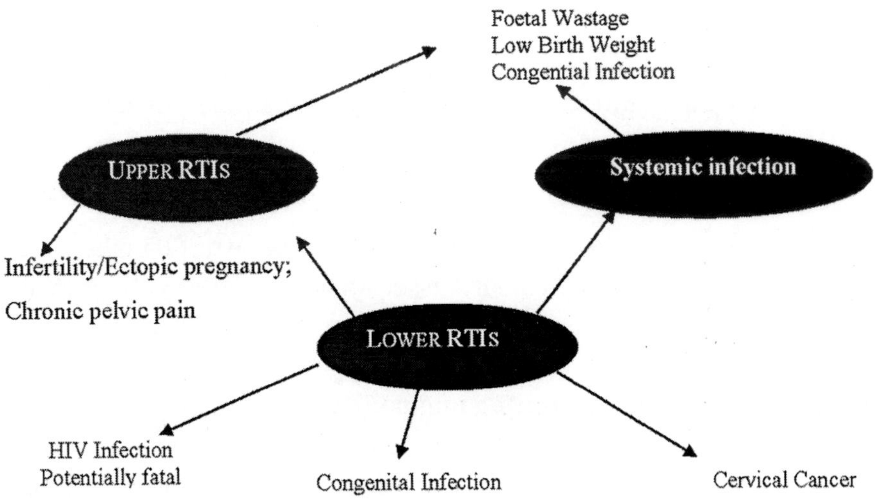

Source: *Wasserheit, J.N. 1992*

Figure 2.1: Sequeale of RTI's

RTI's result in numerous serious consequences. Women suffering from RTI's experience numerous short term biological consequences like vaginal discharge, painful intercourse (dyspaerunia), lower abdominal pain, backache, prolapse, infertility besides facing emotional distress (Wasserheit, 1991). In severe cases RTI may result in cervical cancer, peritonitis, ectopic pregnancy and AIDS. An overview of the consequences of RTI's points to the fact that either directly or through the development of upper genital tract or systemic infection, lower RTI cause numerous potentially devastating sequeale contrary to the general impression that RTI's are not fatal.

An RTI which affects the external genital area such as vulva, vagina and cervix are referred to as lower reproductive tract infection. The migration of infections in the uterus, fallopian tubes and ovaries are considered to be upper reproductive tract infection. RTI's generally originate from the lower reproductive tract i.e. vulva, vagina and cervix. If left untreated, they may ascend to the upper reproductive tract i.e. uterus, fallopian tubes and ovaries to cause pelvic inflammatory disease (PID). This can result in chronic abdominal pain, ectopic pregnancy, menstrual irregularities and infertility as a result of scarring of the fallopian tubes. Thus, lower reproductive tract infection has the propensity of causing lower reproductive tract infection.

Lower RTI's can be broadly classified into three sections on the basis of site of infection:

1. Genital ulcer and lesions: syphilis genital herpes, chancroid and genital warts.
2. Vaginal infection: bacterial vaginosis, candidiasis and trichomoniasis.
3. Cervical infection: Chlamydia and gonorrhea (Wasserheit, 1992).

The upper reproductive tract infection comprise of PID which can also occur asymptomatic but usually associated with lower abdominal pain or tenderness in abdomen, pain or tenderness during pelvic examination when the cervix is touched, unusual vaginal discharge, fever with or without nausea and pain during intercourse. This condition prevails when infection in lower reproductive tract like bacterial vaginosis (Eschenbach, 1993), chlamydia and gonorrhea (Mardh, 1980) remain untreated. The infection, if remain unattended for a certain duration, will ascend towards the upper reproductive tract i.e. uterus, fallopian tubes and the ovaries. This ascendance of infection from the lower to the upper tract is often facilitated by introduction of instruments through the cervix during poor quality medical procedures such as while inserting an intra uterine device (IUD) during procedures such as sterilization or unsafe abortion and delivery practices. Brabin *et al.* in his study on PID in India suggested female sterilization operations conducted in non sterile conditions as a risk factor for PID (Brabin et al., 1992).

In non-pregnant women, the complications of pelvic inflammatory disease (PID) are frequent and usually irreversible. PID results in infertility (via total or partial occlusion of the fallopian tubes due to post inflammatory scarring), ectopic pregnancy and chronic pelvic pain. The incidence of PID caused infertility in developing countries is higher because PID treatment is usually delayed for insufficient duration is completely unavailable. It has been suggested that PID following induced abortion, post partum infection and IUD insertions results in higher tubal occlusion rates and sterility than other types of PID (Westrom and Mardh, 1975). Chronic pelvic pain and recurrent infections too develop among women who have had pelvic infection. Long term sequeale of RTI's include cervical cancer and transmission of HIV virus which is lethal for women.

In pregnant women, both sexually transmitted and endogenous pathogens may play a role in foetal wastage, low birth weight and congenital infection. These complications occur via intra uterine exposure due to upper tract or systemic infection or in the case of congenital infection via exposure to lower tract pathogens during delivery (Wasserheit J.N. 1992). Women with acute chlamydial or gonococcal infection are 3 to 5 times as likely to deliver a low birth weight or premature infant as are uninfected women.

2.4 CLINICAL ASPECTS OF COMMON VAGINAL INFECTIONS

The vagina creates its own environment and maintains a balance among the normal bacteria found there and the hormonal change in a woman's body which is associated with medication such as antibiotics, hormone, vaginal medication, sexual intercourse, STD, stress and change in sexual partner. Vaginal infections or vaginitis describes the most common medical concerns women have in the area of their reproductive organ. It is the inflammation of the vagina that creates discharge odor, irritation or itching. Some of the common infections are Bacterial vaginosis: Candidiasis, Trichomoniasis, Gonorrhea, Chlamydia etc. Bacterial vaginosis is caused when the bacteria normally found in the vagina (Lacto *bacillus*) are overgrown by others e.g. Garderella *vaginalis*. Bacterial vaginosis causes an abnormal vaginal discharge with an unpleasant odor. Some women reported a strong fishlike smell, especially after intercourse. The discharge is usually white or gray. It can be thin. It is also associated with burning during urination or with itching around the outside of the vagina or both. Some women with Bacterial vaginosis have no symptom at all. Bacterial vaginosis can be treated by giving antibiotics in cream gel or tablet form.

Another type of vaginal infection is candidiasis which causes a thick, whitish gray "cottage cheese" type of vaginal discharge and may be itchy. One may have intense itching at the genital region. Painful urination and pain during intercourse are common. It may not always be associated with vaginal discharge. Candidiasis, referred to as thrush or a yeast infection, is caused by the fungus candida. The reason for developing of this infection is not well understood. However, recent use of antibiotics, oral contraceptives that contain progesterone, or the presence of other conditions such as diabetes, pregnancy, or immune suppression can also increase a woman's chances of developing candidiasis. The signs observed by clinician are white, thick curd like discharge, redness of vulva, vaginal and cervical tissue.

Trichomoniasis is another infection caused by a protozoan (a form of parasite) called Trichomonas vaginalis which is transmitted during sex. Trichomoniasis causes a frothy vaginal discharge that may be yellow-green or gray, itching and irritation of genitals, burning during urination (sometimes confused with urinary tract infection), discomfort during intercourse and a foul smell. The medicine for treatment of Trichomoniasis is antibiotic metronidazole.

Chlamydia is caused by sexually transmitted bacterium Chlamydia *trachomatis*. It produce no symptom in women however chlamydia can cause pain while passing urine, long term pelvic pain and infertility. Antibioties like deoxycycline, erythromycin and azithronycin are given by chlamydial treatment.

Gonorrhea: The bacterium responsible for it is Neisseria *gonorrhoea*. The symptoms associated with gonorrhoea are vaginal discharge, pain while passing urine but there may be no symptom in early stage. However, if they are left untreated, it leads to pelvic infection and a general feeling of being unwell.

Infections causes of vaginitis:

Condition	*Standard Clinical & Laboratory Signs*
Candida	Abnormal curd-like discharge, Fungi on wet preparation slide with 10% Potassium Hydroxide (KOH);pH usually < 4.5
Bacterial Vaginosis	**The Amsel Criteria:** A positive diagnosis is made if 3 of the following 4 criteria are present: Speculum examination shows homogeneous vaginal discharge "Clue cells" are found on microscopy (>20%) Vaginal pH> 4.5 A "fishy" odor is produced when 10% Potassium Hydroxide is added to vaginal secretions
Trichomonas infection	Motile, bi-flagellated trichomonads seen on microscopy Frothy discharge; pH usually > 4.5

2.5 THEORETICAL FRAMEWORK

Many theories were developed to explain health outcomes with the implicit assumption that disease symptoms are ubiquitous, viewing health solely as biomedical state. However, Mishler (1981), adumbrated this assumption of biomedical model as the "assumption of generic disease" and defies the assumption that disease symptoms are expected to be similar in different culture and societies during any historical period (Mishler, 1981). To drive home the point that different culture has different perception of disease, Nichter (1989), focus on the examination of "disease" in the context of culture. For this study women's ill health will be examined through the kaleidoscope of biomedical model as well as its cultural construction as an illness. Following are the theoretical framework which will be in use for this study.

2.5.1 Determinants of Reproductive Morbidity:

The main interest of this study is to diagnose the magnitude of the problem of reproductive morbidity. Hence, a panoramic view of the problem covering the process of production of ill-health at the community level and attempt to represent it through a determinants structure is essential. Understanding the determinant and their mechanism for production of the level of ill health is the necessary first step for a realistic policy aimed at alleviating condition of reproductive morbidity.

In analyzing the determinants of various conditions of ill health in population groups, layered approach gave birth. Zurayk et al. (1993), proposed a framework of the determinants of reproductive morbidity borrowing from "layered" approach developed by Davis and Blake (1956) and Bongaarts (1978).

In early 50's an approach originated to examine the determinants of fertility in the work of Davis and Blake (1956) and of Bongaarts (1978). It was introduced into the International public health arena through the work of Mosley and Chen (1984), in an attempt to synthesize in one model the medical and socio-economic determinants of child survival. The approach divides determinants into two categories:

1. The "immediate variables" which have a biological link to the outcome variable of interest; and
2. The "background variables" which operate through the intermediate variable.

Because the immediate variables are more direct in their effect they have alternately been called as the proximate determinants. The background variables represent the social context of ill health. The key to this framework is the identification of a set of proximate determinants or intermediate variables that directly influence the risk of morbidity and mortality. All social and economic determinants operate through these variables to affect the survival of child. The proximate determinants has five factors namely maternal factors, environmental factor, nutrient deficiency, injury and personal illness counted while the background variable include individual level factor, household level factor and community level factor.

Further developments in the framework have added on additional set of factors between the immediate ones and morbidity. Winikoff (1987), in her work on reproductive health and Norren and Vianen (1986), introduced medical risk factors more proximate than the intermediate variables. Thus medical risk was filtered out from the immediate category emphasizing more "proximate" association to an outcome.

On the other hand, the vague expression of the background variables generated concern for the need to open the black box and clarify the important elements in the open the black box and clarify the important elements in the social context of ill health. (Shorter, 1987). Caldwel and Caldwel (1991), showed more concern with the social context and formed the main substance of "health transition" research which is taken to involve the cultural, social and behavioural determinants of health: that is those determinant other than medical interventions. An attempt by Zurayk et al. (1993) to encompass these health transition variables in a theoretical framework of the determinants of general health status provides a rich presentation of both proximate and background factor giving due consideration to structural determinants of health.

Campbell and Graham (1990), Fathalla (1991) and Mc Carthy and Maine (1992), applied layered approach to construct a determinant structure for outcomes concerned with various dimensions of women's reproductive health. Using these existing frameworks as the platform Zurayk et al. (1993), designed a framework to examine the determinants of women's reproductive morbidity.

The framework constructed by Zurayk et al. (1993), comprises of three main blocks: background, intermediate and medical risk factors which affect morbidity. The medical risk factors are considered to be the general health condition or the susceptibility status of a woman. Susceptibility is affected by exposure to nutritional, infections and other morbidities. These are linked together and with reproductive morbidity in a cumulative and interactive fashion (Winikoff, 1988).

Imtermediate variables include a women's childbearing pattern, her use of health services and her health related practices that affect susceptibility. A woman's childbearing pattern relates to her age at the extent of birth spacing. The extent of women's use of health services during pregnancy, at the time of delivery and in the post partum period is also an essential factor in avoiding most of the complication and health hazards associated with childbearing and treating them quickly when they occur. Her utilization of gynecological and general health care is equally important in controlling reproductive morbidity and will depend on her perception of need as well as on availability and especially on quality of services.

A woman's health related behaviours particularly during an episode of pregnancy affect the likelihood of her suffering from reproductive morbidity. Among the important behaviours influencing reproductive health are a woman's diet, her workload and her personal hygiene practices. In terms of RTI a woman's sexual activity or her husband's are important.

The background variables include the personal resources of the women such as education, her urban or rural origin and her work experience. It also include household resources representing the personal resource of the other members of the household particularly the women's husband, as well as housing condition and amenities available. Besides the community resources such as accessibility to health services and individual in contact with health institution, and the support network that women can resort to in health related matters are also important. Finally, the social institution resources, particularly represented by the dominant values related to reproduction and reproductive health care in the community. Although the general direction of this framework is the influence from the determinants to reproductive morbidity condition, it should be noted that reproductive morbidity has severe influence of its own affecting susceptibility, the intermediate factors and some of the background resources.

An illness episode affects a women's general health status and some of her living conditions and behaviour. It is in fact fear of such influence that makes some women endures a condition in silence, rather than change some behaviour, such as workload, that would have detrimental consequences to her position in the household.

The biomedical determinant framework of reproductive morbidity has certain significant hiatus to guide the social science researcher. The people's perception of disease does not fit anywhere in the determinant framework.

Mosley and Chen (1984), mentioned the influence of beliefs about disease causation at an individual level "background" factor Zurayk et al. (1993), empirically tested their framework in Giza, Egypt in studying the reproductive morbidity of women and emphasized the importance of cultural perception of disease or perceived morbidity ratiocination on following points: First, women's health behaviour, particularly in seeking health care is governed by what woman perceive as ill-health whether this perception is consistent with medical symptom or not. Secondly, learning about morbidity as perceived by women brings to attention what worries women about their health based on criteria of seriousness such as discomfort or interference with their daily routines or with the feelings of dignity.

Determinants of Reproductive Morbidity:

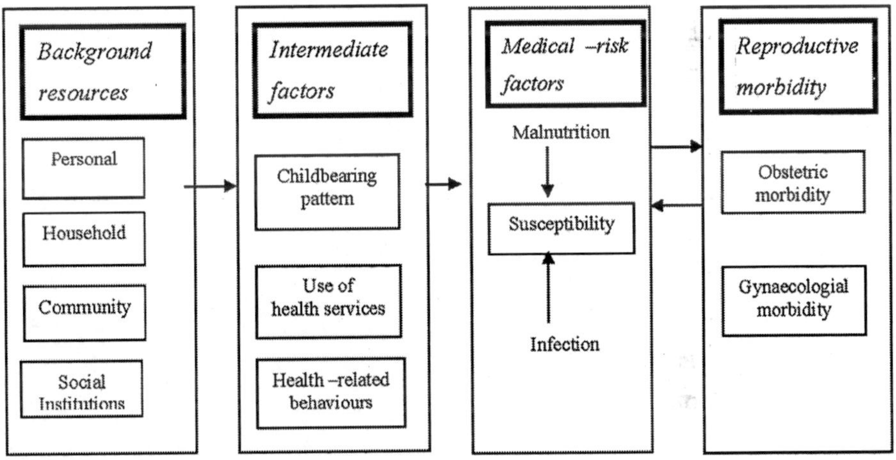

Source: Zurayk et al., 1993

Figure 2.2: Determinants of Reproductive Morbidity

This study is concerned with discussing the policy about the diagnosis of reproductive health and assessment of its determinant and it utilizes the above framework to develop appropriate determinant variables. However, women's perception of reproductive health is centrifocal to this study's objective in demonstrating the relationship between women's perception of morbidity and morbidity itself which is shaped by society's cultural construction of ill health. In continuation to this issue, presented below are different social science perspectives which guided the research on perceptions of reproductive health which is the central focal point of the present study.

2.5.2 Explanatory Model of Reproductive Morbidity:

The study of socio-cultural context of reproductive morbidity can be approached from at least two overlapping and equally important perspectives. In the first, the emphasis is on ethno medical aspects of illness, including belief about diet, body and health, systems of healing, belief about symptoms, causes and consequences (Kleinman, 1980).

Kleinman (1980), proposed a framework which shows the interaction of patients and healers in the context of culture. He proposes that just as each patient operates in his/her cultural system, so do allopathic providers operate within a biomedical cultural system. Perception of the existence of a disease is not a simple recognition of a physical symptom. A man's disease becomes significant only when it is identified as illness, a physiological malfunctioning that is seen to threaten the individual and his society. Societies define illness in different fashions and symptoms that are accepted as evidence of illness in one society may be ignored in another. Kleinman distinguishes between disease which is a biological condition and illness which is a social recognition of a condition. Kleinman referred to this framework as the "explanatory model framework" which he defined as:

Explanatory models are the notion about an episode of sickness and their treatments that are employed by all those engaged in the clinical process. Explanatory models are held by patients and practitioners in all health care systems. They offer explanation of sickness and treatment to guide choices among available therapies and therapists and to cast personal and social meaning on the experience of sickness (Kleinman, 1980).

This theoretical framework demonstrates the relationship between the patient's explanatory model (EM) of an illness and the health care professionals exhibiting cultural competence through developing an understanding of the patient's explanatory model. An explanatory model is constructed to seek answers of etiology, time and mode of onset of symptoms, pathophysiology, course of sickness and treatment (Kleinman, 1980).

According to EM, each patient coming to the practitioner is faced with perspectives and ideas about the illness. It is only through limiting the patient to share his/her explanatory model that the practitioner is able to understand the clients perspective, honour the meaning and care for the patient in a way that respect his/her way of living. Thus, Kleinman emphasizes the importance of EM while considering a health problem because patient and provider's EM differ at levels of analytical power, abstraction, logical articulation, metaphor and idiom. These differences finally lead to therapeutic options and treatment which are different for the patients and provider (Kleinman, 1980).

Explanatory model provides a guide to determine ethno medical model and to compare them to biomedical models in the context of a particular culture. Thus, individuals draw on the ethno medical model of an illness construct an EM when they experience a particular illness episode. Ethno-medical models for reported symptoms like *sarir bahar aave* (Prolapse) among women in rural Rajasthan is different from the biomedical model of prolapse (Oomman, 1996). Consequently, this difference will lead to inaccurate diagnosis and treatment of RTI in the area. By situating a problem at high prevalence of reproductive tract infections by Indian women within this framework, this study proposes to elucidate both the overlap and the hiatus between the two models.

The prime objective of this study is to document women's experience of gynecological complaints through cultural reasoning. Women's EM about what ailed them, levels of concerns associated with persistent complaints, interpretation of symptoms and the progression of illness, forms of self treatment, and patterns of health care seeking as well as the types and quality of health services available to women will be examined.

Though the EM can be employed to determine ethno-medical model and to compare it with biomedical model in the context of culture, its lacunae is that it cannot determine ethno medical model in the context of physical environment and socio-economic condition. To make an end of such situation the ecological framework (Mc Elroy and Townsend, 1989) and the critical medical anthropology perspective (Singer, 1989) are taken up to provide a broader framework and to contain the approach of this research study.

2.5.3 Medical, Ecological and Critical Medical Anthropological Approach:

McElroy and Townsend necessitates to look at health and illness as part of a set of physical, biological and cultural subsystems that continually affect each other. The medical ecological approach (McElroy and Townsend, 1989) links biomedicine with biological and cultural anthropology, resulting in important contribution to the understanding of health and disease as dynamic, adaptive population-based processes. The ecological model is constructed on three key assumptions:

1. There is no single cause of disease; rather, disease is ultimately due to a chain of factors related to ecosystem imbalances.
2. Health and disease are part of a set of physical, biological, cultural subsystem that continually affects one another.
3. The ecological model provides a framework for the study of health in environmental context but does not specify what factors maintain health within any given local system.

On the other hand, critical medical anthropology raises important questions about the impact of political and economic structures and processes on health and disease. (Baer, Singer and Susser, 1997). They focus on health care systems in terms of how they function at multiple levels, including

(a) The individual level of patient experience.

(b) The micro level of physician-patient relationship.

(c) The intermediate level of local health care system, particularly hospitals and clinics.

(d) The macro social level of global political-economic system.

At all these levels, the goal is to understand how existing social relations structure the relationships among the participants in the systems. This is particularly relevant in India where the socio-political context greatly influences a women's capacity to access health care for health problem related to sexual behaviour. This study will explore the reproductive health of women in Manipur guided with a conglomeration of framework which includes elements of ethno-medical model and biomedical model.

2.6 EPIDEMIOLOGY OF GYNECOLOGICAL MORBIDITIES INCLUDING RTI's

The epidemiology of RTI points to a number of risks factors that contribute to the burden of gynecological morbidity. These include sexual behaviour, number of pregnancies, abortion, delivery conditions, contraceptive use and menstrual hygiene (Jejeebhoy and Koenig, 2002; Padian et al. 1991). Underlying these factors are the socio cultural contexts in which many risk behaviours occur (Aral and Wasserheit, 1998). In their framework, Zurayk et al. (1993), showed that socio cultural variables including women's status forms a set of background determinants of gynecological morbidity. They emphasize the need for elaborating the background variables in the light of the importance of power relations in determining the occurrence of gynecological morbidity.

Research in the 1990's has established the significance of reproductive tract infections (RTI) among women in India through community based prevalence studies on gynecological morbidity (Bang et al., 1989; Bhatia et al., 1997). In other developing countries such as Nigeria, Bangladesh and Egypt (Brabin et al., 1995; Wasserheit et al., 1989; Younis et al., 1993) there have been raised awareness among researchers and policy makers, of magnitude of reproductive tract infections and their grave consequence among women.

Due to lack of awareness, fear of social stigmatization and poor access to appropriate services even symptomatic women often fail to seek timely care. Women also tend to suffer more because of the synergistic effects of infection, malnutrition and reproduction. The consequences of untreated RTI's in women range from acute distress to death (Elias, 1991). Among women in India, endogenous and iatrogenic infections contribute significantly to the high prevalence of RTI's. Community based studies among women in different parts of the country report a prevalence of bacterial vaginosis and candidiasis ranging from 14 percent to 62 percent and 1 percent to 34 percent respectively. (Oomman, 1996; Bang et al., 1989; Bhatia et al., 1997; Aggarwal et al., 1999; Nandan et al., 2001; Garg et al., 2002). Studies indicate an association between the role of poor genital/personal hygiene and symptoms of RTI's (Bhatia and Cleland, 1995; Oomman, 1996). Among the iatrogenic causes of infection, the use of IUD has been reported to be a significant risk factor for pelvic inflammatory diseases in some clinic based studies (Shrikande et al., 1995; Shrikande et al., 1998). Sterilized women are more likely to report experiencing lower or upper RTI's compared to non-users or users of reversible contraceptive methods (Bhatia and Cleland, 1995; Oomman, 1996) Studies also report that women who have undergone invasive surgical procedure including dilation and curettage are more likely to experience PID (Gogate et al., 1998).

2.6.1 Global Scenario:

In a community based study in rural area of Bangladesh carried out by Wasserheit (1989) 68 percent of women were found to be suffering from RTI's. Amongst symptomatic women, 2 percent were infected with chlamydia, 35 percent had bacterial vaginosis and 0.4 percent was positive for gonorrhea and 5 percent for trichomoniasis.

Younis et al. (1993), studied the gynecological and related morbidities in rural Egypt among 509 ever married non-pregnant women and found high prevalence of prolapse. In this study by an interdisciplinary team of anthropologists, statisticians and physicians 91.4 percent of women participated in the clinical phase of the study in the two villages. Rigorous methodology was followed by this study team. In a sample of 509 women, 83 percent of women had vaginal or cervical discharge at the time of clinical examination. Laboratory testing of discharge were conducted on 44 percent of women who were diagnosed as having vaginitis during clinical examination. Trichomoniasis and bacterial vaginosis was more predominantly prevalent then yeast infections. 10 percent of women were diagnosed having cervicitis during clinical observation. Laboratory results showed chlamydial infection in 86 percent of women and "non-specific" cervicitis in about 9 percent of women. Only 2 percent had definite PID (Uterine tenderness +/- adnexal tenderness) and cervicitis while about 17 percent were diagnosed as "possible" PID (uterine tenderness only). Cervical ectopy was found in about 22 percent of women, while 8 percent had cervical cell changes. About 56.4 percent of women had at least one form of genital prolapse (Younis et al., 1993). Related morbidities like anemia, hypertension, obesity and syphilis were also found which reveal an extremely high incidence of gynecological morbidity among rural Egyptian women.

The study showed that presence of uterine prolapse with or without vaginal prolapse, availability of husband and IUD use are positive predictors for infection. Predictors for prolapse were found to be associated with age and number of deliveries. This study not only pointed out levels of infection and possible risk factors but also compared women's reported symptoms with disease demonstrating an overall poor agreement of symptom reports with infection, particularly for vaginal discharge (Zurayk et al., 1995). However, as the researchers have pointed out, the study did not examine women's perceptions of their illnesses for better understanding of the meanings of the symptoms they reported (Zurayk et al., 1993).

In another study by Brabin, Kemb and Obunge (1995), among the adolescent girls in rural Nigeria undertaken to determine the rate of prevalence of RTI's, a total of 868 women were interviewed and examined of which 458 were aged 21 and above and 410 were aged between 12-19 years. Amongst adolescents below 17 years of age, 19.8 percent had candida and 11.1 percent had trichomonas infections. In the age group 17-19 years chlamydia was detected in 10.5 percent, candidiasis in 25.6 percent and 43.8 percent had any infection. Overall, 42.1 percent of sexually active adolescents had experienced either an abortion or STD.

2.6.2 RTI in the Indian Domain

The extent of RTI's among women in India remains to be a moot issue. Much of the available data was limited to high risk or clinic - based populations and indicated a relatively high prevalence of many RTI's. Reports of men and women attending government sexually transmitted disease (STD) clinics, points to an increasing trend in the number of cases seen at the clinics, from 1981 to 1991. (Luthra et al., 1992). The actual numbers are likely to be an underestimate, largely because substantial number of cases resort to private practitioner or pharmacies for treatment and therefore go unreported. Furthermore, no large surveys have been conducted at a national level to ascertain the prevalence of STD's and other RTI's (Luthra et al., 1992).

In the last few years, a number of community based prevalence studies of gynecological morbidity among women have been undertaken in India. The findings provided invaluable insights into the problem of gynecological morbidity in general and RTI's in particular.

The community based study carried out by Bang and Bang in rural Maharastra was an eye opener for various researchers. 650 women were studied of which 55 percent had gynecological complaints and 92 percent of women had one or more gynecological examination and treatment. The study showed prevalence of 14 percent for trichomoniasis, 34.1 percent for candidiasis, 62 percent of bacterial vaginitis and 115 for syphilis (Bang and Bang, 1989).

Another community based study carried out in Alipur by the Department of Community Medicine; Maulana Azad Medical College demonstrated that 77 percent of women had gynecological complaints. Cytological smears revealed presence of inflammation (62 percent) trichomonas vaginalis (7 percent) candida (0.4 percent) and condyloma (0.7 percent). The prevalence of moderate dysplasia or malignancy in this setting was 0.2 percent (Oomman, 1996).

A survey of 370 female sex workers in West Bengal revealed that 13.2 percent of these women were suffering from gonorrhea, 58.8 percent from syphilis, 11.1 percent from trichomoniasis and 23.2 percent from candidiasis (Singh, 1995). In all, 80.6 percent of these women were infected with single or multiple RTI pathogens.

Community based studies conducted in rural as well as urban areas of India namely Maharastra, West Bengal, Mumbai, Gujarat and Kerala to assess the levels of reported and clinically assessed gynecological morbidity show high level of infection. Gynecological morbidity measured by clinical examination revealed that vaginitis was found ranging from 4 percent to 62 percent, cervicitis in 85 to 48 percent PID in 1 percent to 24 percent and genital prolapse in 0.5 percent to 18 percent. The variation in level of morbidity should be considered on the basis that study populations were different and the difference in diagnostic criteria for morbidities.

A study by Bhatia and Cleland (1995) among the rural women in Karnataka highlighted that one third of all women reported at least one symptom of gynecological morbidity and one tenth of women having sexually transmitted disease comprising of trichomonas vaginalis (75 percent) gonorrhea (0.8 percent), syphilis (1.5 percent) and candidiasis (5.2 percent). According to their findings, sterilized women are more likely to report morbidity as compared to users of contraceptive methods. Reporting of symptoms was also less among women who delivered in private institutes as compared to those who delivered in government hospitals.

2.6.3 Correspondence between Perception and Diagnosis:

A growing concern in reproductive health is the conflicting data available which compares self-reported reproductive morbidity with clinical and/or laboratory diagnosis of reproductive morbidity. Some studies have higher rates of clinical or laboratory diagnosed morbidity (Bang, 1989; Bhatia, 1999) while others have higher rates of self reported morbidity (Bhatia and Cleland, 2000). In fact, findings drawn from different sources - self reports, clinical examination and laboratory testing are often inconsistent and only in exceptional circumstances, is there likely to be a correlation between self reported and medically diagnosed morbidities. As such, it becomes increasingly difficult to evaluate reproductive morbidity within any population using one methodology (Khanna, 2001).

Oomman (1996) in her study in a Rajasthan village had correlated vaginal discharge as a symptom with gynaecologist examination and laboratory investigation. Of 250 women, 78.8 percent reported of *dhola pani* (discharge), 19.6 percent of prolapse. 194 women who reported of discharge were examined by gynaecologist and 131 women were identified having discharge. The symptoms were found to be 85.5 percent sensitive and 28.7 percent specific. The reported symptoms of discharge were also compared with the gynaecologist's diagnosis of either vaginitis/cervicitis. The positive predictive value showed that symptoms (47.9 percent) predicted the presence of any RTI. 52.8 percent agreement with a kappa of 0.12 indicated that there was moderate concordance between women's symptoms and signs. Comparison of symptom with laboratory investigation revealed poor agreement (PPV 16.1 percent, agreement 31.6 percent and Kappa = 0.002). Clinical diagnosis of lower RTI showed moderate concordance with laboratory infection.

To surmise, these studies strongly indicate high level of gynecological level although there is variation in level from one region to another. Thus, generalization cannot be made for other parts of India. Only one of these studies (Oomman, 1996) emphasize in understanding reproductive morbidity through the cultural meanings. Oomman work jotted the women's perceptions about their body anatomy and physiology and related it to the symptom they report. This study compares women's reported symptom with medically diagnosed condition, and examined the socio-economic, environmental and economic determinants of gynecological morbidity, their treatment seeking behaviour and source of information and advice for gynecological problems.

It is evident from the above review that RTI form a heavy burden in India and are responsible for a significant amount of female morbidity. The actual numbers are likely to be more as majority remain unreported. This increasing trend calls for an urgency for developing need based interventions.

3

Research Methods

This chapter reflects on one year field work in Andro and Kwakeithel which was a unique first hand experience. I had to adopt certain strategies compatible with the situation or condition of my field area. Besides the methods that are scripted out in books a researcher has to scoop out her natural skill in establishing rapport and extracting information. It also discusses the procedures used to protect the identity of the informant and to maintain confidentiality of the information revealed to the researcher as well as limitations of the study.

3.1 CHOICE OF THE STUDY AREA

These areas were chosen because it follows certain criteria:

1. Andro is a typical rural area while Kwakeithel is a peri-urban community in terms of its location and economic activities. For Kwakeithel, eight localities were selected which goes in congruence with the definition of peri-urban.
2. Proximity and accessibility: Andro is just 26 kms. away from Imphal and there is bus service to and fro.
3. Andro was the field area for my M. Phil. Dissertation which enable me to have an already established rapport with the families in Andro ensuring an easy access to information. Establishing rapport in both the areas was not an issue.

For field-work, I stayed in one of the household in Andro which saved my time and energy in traveling up and down from Andro to Imphal. Moreover, staying and living in their midst helped me more in understanding their life and establishing a good rapport with the people.

As an anthropologist, I started for my sojourn in Andro as a field worker in July 2004 and for Kwakeithel in January 2005. The study was cross-sectional in design and conducted in three phases:

(i) Ethnographic

(ii) Survey and

(iii) Clinical.

In this chapter I will endeavor to present the different components of data collection and management in each of the three phases of the study.

3.2 ETHNOGRAPHIC PHASE

This phase of the study was undertaken from July to August 2004 in Andro and from January to February in Kwakeithel. The purpose of this phase was-

(a) To develop an understanding of the socio-economic and cultural context in which women in Andro and Kwakeithel experience, define and express their lives;

(b) To elicit local terminology regarding women's illnesses;

(c) To construct an ethno-medical model i.e. causes, progression and health seeking behaviour of women's reproductive illnesses to help devise structured data collection instrument. Each woman was visited at her house and detailed history regarding identification data, socio-demographic profile, menstruation and related disorder, obstetric history and related morbidity, infertility, reproductive morbidity health seeking behavior, contraception behavior was obtained or recorded. History relating to present reproductive morbidity, or that, which has occurred within last six months, was also taken.

To investigate the key issues of my research, holistic approach was used. Both qualitative as well as quantitative methods were triangulated to investigate different aspects of reproductive health. Besides, to brush up the various dimensions of women's reproductive morbidity, initially unstructured questionnaire were used to collected data in order to establish key topics, which were later on followed by semi-structured methods.

3.2.1 Village Mapping:

Village mapping was used to construct the map of Andro village. Experience in India has shown that this is a very useful technique to obtain an accurate map of a village (Gittelsohn et al., 1995). Village people have a vivid idea of locations in their surroundings. This session was conducted using pen, pencil and paper so that it could be retained for further use. This method was carried out with a group of men and women and facilitated me the whereabouts in the village. This map served as a guide for the survey phase. It furnishes me information about the location of market, temple, lake, health center, small shops in the village, village school, etc. Andro is quite a large village but they could locate everything in every nook and corner of the village.

3.2.2 Focus Group Discussion:

The benefits of focus group discussion are well recognized in particular the opportunity they afford to the researcher to observe group participants interacting and recounting specific views, opinions, attitudes and experiences (Berg, 1998). Focus group discussions do not discriminate against those who are illiterate. They also encourage participation from people reluctant to be interviewed on their own or who feel they have nothing to say (Kitzenger, 1995). Focus group can generate large amount of data in relatively short span of time.

The principal aim during the focus group discussion with women was to develop an understanding of women's perception of normal against abnormal reproductive tract symptoms (such as vaginal or urethral discharge), infectious against non-infectious condition and their explanation of the ways in which

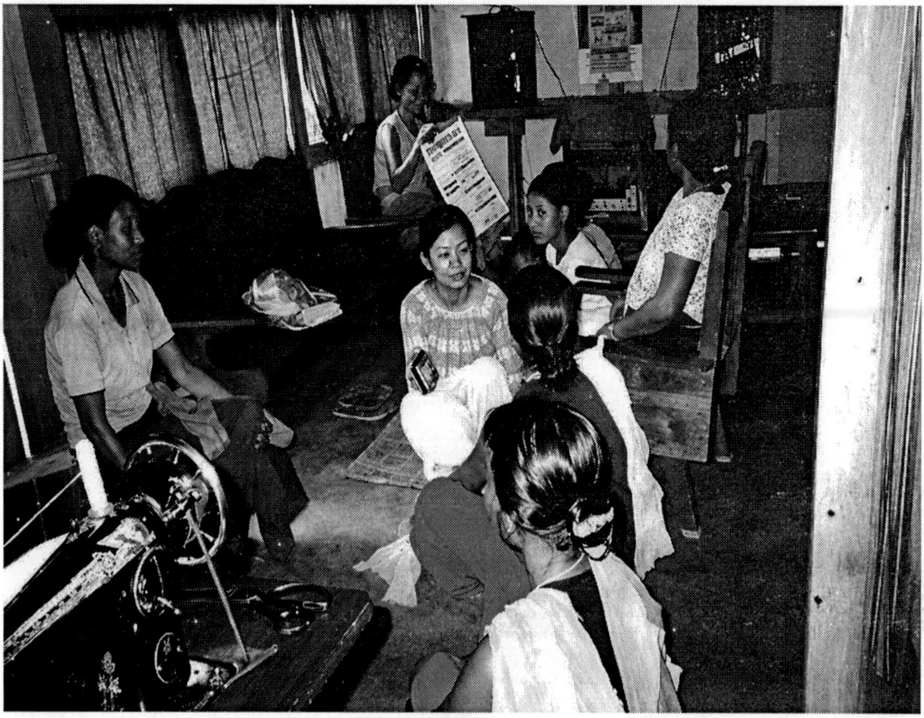

Figure 3.1: Focus Group Discussion Session.

women acquire, prevent or deal with such a condition. Special attention was paid to the association of these perceptions with traditional belief about illness and healing, as well as the perceived accessibility and quality of family planning and reproductive health services. Emphasis was devoted to understand decisions affecting coital debut and the acquisition and development of knowledge concerning reproductive health. Exploration of perceived interaction between reproductive tract morbidity and various contraceptive method, the wisdom and feasibility of advocating reproductive tract infection prevention were covered up in the focus group discussion. Discussion on perceived impact of pregnancy and postpartum period on reproductive tract infection symptoms and morbidity were also touched. Attention was also given to the issues of self treatment and sexual abstinence during symptomatic period and changes in male sexual behavior during symptomatic period and changes in male sexual behavior during times when they are pregnant or during postpartum period.

Table 3.1: Data Collection Method During Ethnographic Study

Data collection tool	*Target*	*Information collected*	*Number reached*
Village mapping	Group of men and women	Village layout	2
Key important interview	Old women in the community, traditional healers, *maibis*, and primary health centre staff.	Illness, causes, treatment, childbirth, menstruation, sexual behaviour, food taboo, women's works	20
Focus group discussion	Women's groups (Mahila, Mandal, Nisha Bandh, Meira Paibi) Traditional birth attendants (TBA)	Women' illness, treatment, sexual behaviour, foods	6
Body mapping	Women and TBA	Ethno anatomy, ethno physiology, women's illnesses	2
Direct observation	Households, visits to specific health providers, in an around the community.	Local treatments, type of house, amenities	12
Participant observation	Field visits, local medicine shop.	Women's work, local treatments, childbirth	3
Case study	Women in reproductive age group	Women's illness, progression and treatment taken	7
Free listing of illness identified as women's health problem.	Women in reproductive age group	Women's illnesses	6
Check list of illnesses identified as women's health problems	Women in the reproductive age group	Women's illness, symptom, causes, treatments, confidants	10
Past illness narratives	Women identified by local healers as having problem	Causes of illness, progression of illness, treatments sought, confidants	14

Semi-structured Interviews	Local health provider	Treatment for women's illnesses	4

Focus group discussion proved to be a culturally sensitive means of data collection. It was encouraging that people were very open in their discussion of sexual matters. However, there were a number of limitations to be accounted for selection of participants was conducted by informants and was not random. Therefore selection bias cannot be ruled out. Although attempts were made to maintain homogeneity within each group, participants tended to self select into groups of familiarity. In dealing with sensitive issues of sexual health, good rapport was felt to be more important than rigid pre-defined groups according to age and marital status. Another limitation is that participants frequently stated that they had never experienced such infections and often one person would make this statement on behalf of the group. Such a statement of denial many have closed off the possibility of other participants disclosing their personal experiences of having reproductive tract infection and seeking care.

The focus group discussions were tape recorded, translated and transcribed into English and then subjected to qualitative analysis. The data was collected in local dialect i.e. Meiteilon and was later transcribed in English.

3.2.3 Pre-testing:

Pre-testing of the questionnaire was conducted on both Andro and Kwakeithel in July 2004. The questions were tested among 5 females to assess the logistics and suitability. Ambiguous questions were modified or excluded from the final questionnaire. Questions that did not generate any meaningful responses were removed and more direct rather than exploratory were added. The interview technique was geared to be active since it was found that women in the pre-testing questions phase were replying monosyllabically to most of the questions. At the same time, a conscious effort was made to explore the treatment modalities and explanation of the disease provided by the non-allopathic health care provides.

3.2.4 Case Studies:

The case studies were carried out with a view to obtain a more comprehensive understanding of the causality and the socio-cultural context in which reproductive tract infections are acquired, the stages and processes involved in the patterns of treatment seeking behaviors, how and why the infections occurred and how they are perceived and managed by the women and their families.

Information and explanation were sought in relation to the patterns of treatment seeking behaviors and the processes involved in treatment seeking such as their perception of the causality and type of symptoms, the significance of these symptoms, role of home remedies, indigenous and other alternative treatments for specific illness, the sequence and experiences of action taken and consideration such as affordability, role of women's decision making in intra familial context and other influencing factors.

The interview also focused on their perception of the causality of genital infections and illness i.e. the extent to which the symptoms are attributed to the behavior of the husbands, contraceptive use, abortions and possibly their own behaviors that might expose them to risk of infections.

3.2.5 Key Informant Interviews:

Key informant interviews were conducted with the *Maibis* (Traditional Birth Attendant), older women in the community and traditional healers. They were chosen specifically for their knowledge regarding the reproductive health of women in the community. This enabled the researcher to explore the domain of women's health problems by asking informants open ended question and thereafter asserting minimum control over the interview. Topics which emerged from these interviews included different kinds of illnesses in the community: women's illnesses, men's illnesses and children's illnesses, causes for illnesses, women's work pattern, *maibis* (midwives) and child delivery practices, menstruation and menstrual practices, sexual behaviour and hygienic condition.

3.2.6 Body Mapping:

All system of knowledge is socially constructed. Assess to people's knowledge of their bodies from verbal description is difficult. Body mapping (Gittelsohn et al., 1994; Mac Cormack, 1985) was used in graphs to document the ethno-anatomy and ethno-physiology of women's bodies. A body map serves as a template for further discussion about topics like menstruation, pregnancy, childbirth, vaginal discharge and genital prolapse. Body mapping is used to explore issues of desire, sexuality and body image. Body mapping was conducted with group of village women and with a group of *maibi* (midwife). Ordinary village women could not provide detailed description of female anatomy however by providing an outline they consulted with each other about the different parts of the body organs and gave a haphazard sketch of women's physiology. The *maibis* (midwife), on the other hand can provide a better insight regarding the physiology of women. The use of body mapping provided an entry point to explore experiences that might otherwise have been ignored. The completed body map served as an ideal reference point from which women could explain body processes like menstruation or illness like vaginal discharge, prolapse, etc.

3.2.7 Observation Method:

Observation method was employed to gather information on topics related to women's illnesses. Using sensory organ an ethnographer maps the settlement, takes a census of households, describes activities, clothing and other artifacts and notes what people say and do in specific situation (Honingmann, 1959).

3.2.8 Direct Observation:

Direct observation, a technique developed to continuously monitor time and events (Bernard, 1988) was used to document household and field activities of women during the day, activities at health center and traditional healer, to observe household chores of different economic strata in the village and the sanitation, health and hygiene of the people in field area which will be played back later via memory.

3.2.9 Participant Observation:

Participant observation is a process by which one may observe events by not merely observing but also participating in an event itself (Bernard, 1988, Gittelsohn, 1994). I had an opportunity to accompany a *maibi* (midwife) to one childbirth which took place during my stay in Andro. The observation recorded for this method served as a cross-check of delivery practices described by the *maibi* (midwife) verbally and the women earlier in the study. This method was also used to observe a women's work day, leaving and selling of medicine at the local chemist shop, primary health centre services etc. Different types of semi-structured methods were used for different purposes. These methods are very close to unstructured interviews which allow the interviewee to control the interviews, the only different being that the interviewer has an interview guide to ask specific questions in a specific order (Bernard, 1988).

3.2.10 Free Listing:

To get the general perception of women regarding common prevalent illnesses amongst them, free listing technique was used. Free listing is a structured interview technique used to delineate and define a domain. It provided a glossary of illnesses which were considered important by women. It is useful in that it provides information about informant's cognitive structure as they recall items prompted by question (Weller and Romney, 1988). The purpose of this method was to determine the items which make up the domain of illnesses which only women get. Women were randomly chosen for this particular method.

3.2.11 Pile Sorting:

Pile sorting facilitated in providing the combination of diseases which respondents felt were generally linked. These techniques provided the cognitive ideas regarding perception of etiology of illnesses, specific symptoms for illnesses, particular treatments for illnesses, particular treatments for illness and whom women confide when they fall sick.

3.2.12 Past Illness Narrative:

Past illness narrative were used on women who has been identified by *maibi* (midwife) and traditional healer or other women who have particular symptoms like vaginal discharge, menstrual problem, uterine prolapse, etc. Data collected from these interviews were useful in documenting further details of specific illness items within the domain of woman's illnesses. Local terms for these symptoms were also collected and these terms were used to elicit symptom reporting. Illness narrative covers the range of topics in the history of the illness episodes and is also useful in cross checking information. The methodology of obtaining illness episode and probe for details on symptom onset, management and its perceived consequences on their lives can be conveniently covered in illness narrative. Topics also encompass women's marital, reproductive and sexual histories, work patterns etc.

3.2.13 Semi-structured Interviews:

Semi-structured interviews were conducted with local healers to determine if women came to these healers for treatment of women's illnesses.

3.3 SURVEY PHASE

The survey phase was conducted in Andro from September to October 2004 and February to March 2005 in Kwakeithel. The main and reason for conducting survey phase was to measure the determinants of women's reproductive health problems including socio- economic demographic, obstetric and menstrual factors.

Data furnished from the ethnographic phase was used as a springboard to survey phase. The information collected during ethnographic phase was useful in determining the question content and appropriateness of a question. Certain information on topics like household work and earning, household items such as number and type of livestock, house type, obstetric, menstrual and sexual practices within the community was used to develop specific question in the instrument. The instrument was divided into three sections:

(i) *Household, economic situation*: This includes questions like number of family member and their source of income, the number of livestock, household amenities, etc.

(ii) *Household demography*: This section of question tries to highlight information about a woman's family and herself in relation to other household members. This included the name of the woman, her husband's name, head of the household, the woman's position in the family in relation to other women in the family, her age and educational level.

(iii) *Reproductive health component:* Reproductive health components included both open and closed ended questions. This section was designed to procure a woman's obstetric and menstrual history, information about her husband's and her own sexual behavior, current health and reproductive health problem and use of reproductive health services. Specific questions were also asked to determine women's perception, beliefs and practices regarding their own health, reproductive health and related issues in their community.

Collecting data pertaining to household economic situation was the most difficult task. It took quite sometime and it bored respondents most of the time. Questions regarding their current age, education often frustrated the informants.

(i) Data collection procedure:

Reproductive health questionnaire was administered on 200 women aged fifteen and older who were ever married and who live in a particular house as a permanent member and not as a visiting relative or guest. In Andro, there were 675 ever married women between the age of 15 - 45. Since it was impossible to survey the entire Andro village, I took up every third household in Andro from which all available ever married women between the age of 15-45 were interviewed. A household list available in Andro youth club was used to record the houses. For Kwakeithel, the household list was obtained from the deputy commissioner office. For Kwakeithel too women in every third household were taken up for the study. Some houses had to be revisited to interview women who were absent during first visit.

Before the interview begins, the purpose and procedure of the interview was described to the interviewee. Only after obtaining verbal consent from the respondent, the interview is preceded assuring about the confidentiality of the information furnished from her. The interview was conducted in local dialect. The open ended questions were recorded in verbatim.

There are 13 *leikais* (localities) in Andro. To keep track of the household visited, only after all the houses has been visited in one locality I move on to another *leikai* (locality). For Kwakeithel, out of 16 *leikais* (localities), I have taken up *8 leikais* (localities) which can be subsumed under the definition of peri-urban.

3.4 CLINICAL PHASE

The clinical phase was undertaken from October to November 2004 in Andro and from March to April 2005 in Kwakeithel. This was specifically conducted to obtain data to permit a direct comparison of women's perception of their reproductive illnesses with a gynaecologist's description and diagnosis of these illnesses at the time of examination.

There were 13 localities in Andro and two medical health camps were conducted in Andro. In one camp, six localities were informed and in the second camp the remaining seven localities were informed. To inform these women who were interviewed during survey phase, the *meira paibi* president and vice-president were contacted and they in turn sent by words of mouth that health camp will be conducted on a particular date. I did not need to revisit them to inform the informants. Everyone turned up as they had levied fine for absentees. A total of 205 women excluding the unmarried girls came for the clinical examination. However, only 194 women were found valid for this particular study.

In Kwakeithel, the *Nisha bandh* was informed about the free medical health camp. Moreover, announcement was made in and around Kwakeithel through loudspeaker about the health camp. Many women regardless of age turned up as the announcer forgot to mention the age. So, girls having menstrual problem and old women having different ailments come to seek treatment. Free medicine was also distributed which also lured women to attend for free health camp. 210 women turned up for the health camp but unmarried girls and women who are menstruating or pregnant are not included in this study. Only 190 women are valid for this particular study.

3.4.1 Development and Pre-testing of Instruments:

Four different instruments were used in this phase of study.

(i) The survey instrument

(ii) The symptom form was developed specifically to elicit information about three main women's illnesses: *Phingou chatpa* (vaginal discharge), *Mangbaga Mari leinaba anaba* (Problems related with menstruation) *angangkhao nanthaba* (prolapse) which were commonly mentioned by women in the ethnographic phase. This form was reviewed by the gynaecologist. The instrument was tested on 5 women from Andro and another 5 women from Kwakeithel and changes were made in the way questions were phrased and in the order in which they were asked.

(iii) The clinical form was developed by a gynaecologist, who extended a helping hand because she was interested in this particular area. There are five sections ordered according to the examination procedure: (i) abdominal examination (ii) examination of the vulva (iii) speculum examination (iv) bimanual examination. The form includes a section for basic measurements such as height, weight, blood pressure of a woman.

The Laboratory form was developed by the gynaecologist. It included sections for the detection of micro organism such as yeast, bacteria and trichonomas in vaginal discharge smears. It was printed in English only.

3.4.2 Clinical Data Collection:

The gynaecologist who performed the pelvic examination for this study is a trained gynaecologist who was working in Regional Institute of Medical Sciences, Imphal. She was kind enough to spare time to be on the site i.e. Andro and Kwakeithel. Moreover, her keen interest in this topic also helped out. Four other post graduate students from Regional Institute of Medical Science helped her out during health camp which was organized in Andro and Kwakeithel. Another girl, who had completed her course as general nursing, was trained to conduct the symptom and survey interviews. Training for the symptom interview is described below:

(1) Explanation of the objective of the clinical phase.

(2) Obtaining consent from women for the symptom interview and examination after describing the purpose and procedure for both.

(3) Recording all open ended questions exactly as a woman described them.

(4) Signing the form and preparing the woman for the clinical examination.

In Andro, three girls from Andro helped out in boiling the speculum, carrying out the used one and bringing the boiled one and in assisting the gynaecologist in the examination room. In Kwakeithel, relatives gave a helping hand.

3.4.3 Sampling for the Clinical Phase:

The total sample for the whole Andro village comprises of 194 women and for Kwakeithel 190 women who choose to come for a clinical examination. The criteria for a clinical examination were that a woman should be married or was ever married and should be 15 years or older. This was in keeping with the cultural norm that virginal women may not be examined. Initially, only women less than 46 years of age were encouraged to participate. However, several older women who complained of vaginal discharge or prolapse wished to be examined, were also included. If a woman was menstruating and wanted to be examined then she was allowed to but was not included in the final analysis of data. Pregnant woman was also not allowed for examination.

3.4.4 Procedure for clinical examination:

The procedure for clinical examination included eleven steps:

(i) Information Dissemination:

Women from different localities one informed by the *Meira Paibi* members by words of mouth that a lady doctor would visit their particular village on a particular date. On the scheduled day, the Primary health center, Andro was opened and examination started. On the first day, initially few turned up but after few hours women started flocking up as words started spreading out that gynaecologist was examining properly. On the second health camp it was the women who were waiting for the gynaecologist's arrival.

In Kwakeithel, many people turned up starting from the first day. The announcement made on the loudspeaker was effective. Young unmarried girls having menstrual problem also turned up. Old women complaining of weakness backpain etc too came with the hope of getting relief. They were sent to the counter distributing medicine as they were not examined by the gynaecologist.

(ii) Setting up a place for clinical examination:

The site for clinical examination was Andro primary health centre as it was in the epicenter of all the localities. The health camps were conducted only on holidays which were convenient for the gynaecologist and for the primary health centre workers. There were five rooms in primary health centre. The first room was used as registration room and to dispense off medicines. The second room served as physical examination room and women were interviewed before and after clinical examination. The room adjacent to this room was the gynecological examination room. The Andro primary health centre was generous enough for letting me use the microscope, weighing machine and gas stove for boiling the speculums.

For Kwakeithel, the clinical examination room was set up in one club called Pakhangba cultural club. Permission was sought from the club president for organizing free health camp in the club. One room was arranged for examination and the main hall was divided as physical examination room and medicine dispersement room. Within the physical examination room women, were interviewed before and after the examination. The microscope examination was done within the clinical examination room. Two health camp were organized in Kwakeithel and 210 women turned up in total.

To make the examination bed, two tables were joined together. A table was also set up to put the microscope and to make the KOH and saline vaginal discharge preparation.

(iii) Registration:

When a woman came forward to be examined her name, locality, husband's name, head of the household's name were recorded and then she was asked to sign the consent form after reading out the things that were written and that the woman agreed to have a gynecological examination. Each woman was given an identity number which corresponded to the number on her symptom form, clinical form and laboratory form.

(iv) Height, Weight, Hemoglobin and Blood Pressure:

After registration two of them would measure each woman's height weight, blood pressure and hemoglobin level are noted down as records on the clinical form.

(v) Symptom History:

After registration the woman was interviewed about her symptom using the symptom form simultaneously while measuring height, weight, hemoglobin and blood pressure.

(vi) Gynecological examination:

The gynaecologist conducted the examination in four steps: (i) abdominal (ii) vulval (iii) per speculum (iv) per vaginal or biannual. During the per speculum examination she also inserted a pH paper strip in the woman's vagina and took swabs of discharge for further examination. She would smear two glass slides with a swab stick. The microbiologist would immediately prepare the sides for diagnostic test. After the examination the gynaecologist filled in the clinical form and the slide with smears were kept for further laboratory test. *vi) Laboratory test:* On receiving the slide with smears the microbiologist put a drop of KOH on one smear and the other smear is dipped in saline solution for the further laboratory test. Cover slips were placed on them. Laboratory test of Pap smear for 269 women were done in RIMS while 115 were sent to MAMC (Maulana Azad Medical College).

The microbiologist would check for the presence of a fishy odor in the KOH preparation which suggests the presence of gardenella vaginals (Bacterial Vaginosis) in the discharge. This is known as the "Whiff test" and is done as soon as KOH is added to the sample of discharge. The microbiologist carried out the following microscopic test:

(1) Presence of hyphae and spores in the KOH preparation indicating a yeast infection.

(2) Presence of few white blood cells on saline mount, consistent with either baterial vaginosis or candidiasis.

(3) Presence of protozoa or saline mounts indicating the presence of Trichomonas vaginalis in the vaginal discharge sample.

(4) Increased ratio of white cells to as compared to epithelial cells in saline preparation of purulent discharge indicating cervicitis or infection of the cervix.

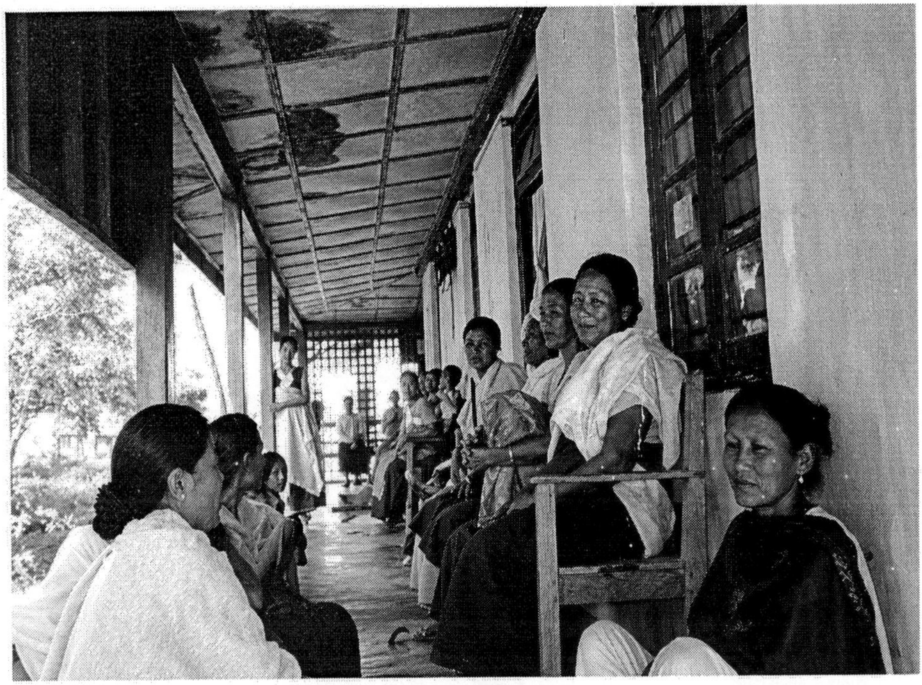

Figure 3.2: Women Waiting for Clinical Examination during Health Camp

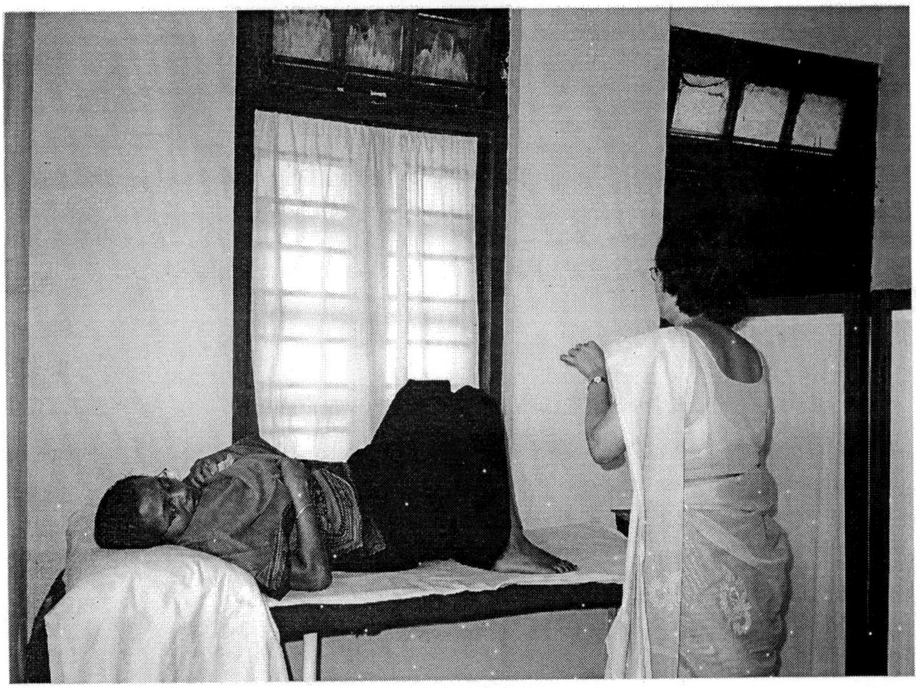

Figure 3.3: Gynaecologist taking Pap Smear

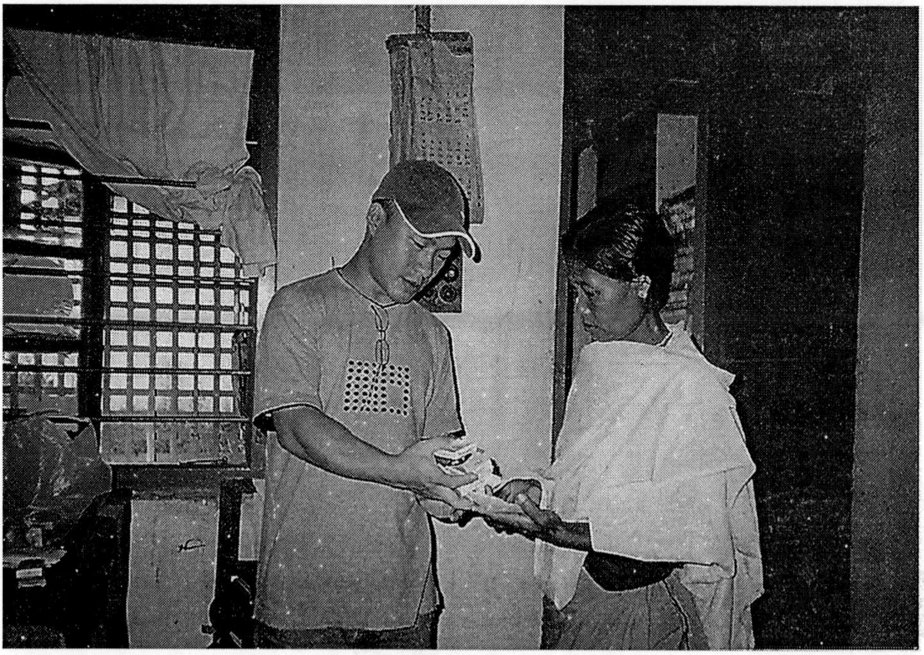

Figure 3.4: Distribution Of Medicine

(vii) Diagnosis Methods:

Diagnosis of a women's gynecological morbidity was made by the gynaecologist on the basis of clinical examination. Major clinical entities were diagnosed as per standard criteria (Stamm W.E. et al., 1988).

(1) *Abnormal discharge*: Complaint and presence of vaginal discharge during examination. The discharge was described in terms of amount, colour, consistency and its association with itching.

(2) *Cervicitis*: Presence of cervical erythema (inflammation) or cervical bleeding on touch with or without discharge.

(3) *Cervical erosion*: A bright red clearly defined area on the vaginal aspect of the cervix where squamous epithelium is replaced by columnar epithelium.

(4) *Pelvic inflammatory disease*: Presence of abdominal tenderness and uterine tenderness, with or without adnexal tenderness.

(5) *Prolapse*: Confirmed by direct examination.

Rectocoele prolapse: Descent of posterior vaginal wall below its normal position.

Cystoesele prolapse: Descent of anterior vaginal wall below its normal position.

Uterine Prolapse: Descent of the uterus below its normal position.

(viii) Treatment, Referral and Follow-up:

A preliminary diagnosis was made based on the clinical examination. Accordingly, women were given medication or were referred to doctors in Regional Institute of Medical Sciences (RIMS)

3.5 ETHICAL CONSIDERATIONS

Ethical procedures were followed at every stage of the study. During ethnographic phase all the interviews were conducted in Meiteilon. The purpose of the interview and the consent form were read to the woman after which the interview was conducted. Attempts were made to conduct the interview in privacy so that respondent could answer question `without any hesitation. All the data collected in this phase are available only to the researcher.

During the survey phase also all the interviews were conducted in Meiteilon local dialect of the area. The purposes of the interview and consent form were read to women before the interview was conducted to obtain her consent. All the information gathered during the survey phase was kept confidential.

For clinical examination, an experienced gynaecologist was hired. Before examination a woman was asked for her consent. The examination was conducted only when the woman agreed. After reading out the consent form they signed it or taken a thumb print. Women were given the option to stop the examination at any moment. The examination is a routine gynecological examination. All instruments were sterilized prior to each examination. All women were treated for current infection at the time of examination and those who required long term treatment were asked to come in Regional Institute of Medical Sciences (RIMS). All the information gathered during the clinical examination phase is confidential and available only to the researcher.

3.6 DATA MANAGEMENT AND DATA ENTRY

Every data collection event was recorded into a note book. The data collected during focus group discussions are recorded in audio tape recordings are later transcribed in English. The data collected were later expanded into notes. The numerically coded data are entered in SPSS 11.0

For comparison of women's self reported symptoms with the clinical and laboratory diagnosis, sensitivity, Specificity, Positive predictive value, Negative predictive value, Agreement, Kappa were calculated.

- *Sensitivity:* Ability of the test to find out correct/positive cases out of actual positive.
- *Specificity:* Ability of the test to find out true negative out of the total people who do not have the case.
- *Positive predictive value:* proportion of true positive among all those who reported phingou chatpa.
- *Negative predictive value:* Proportion of true negative among all those who reported the absence of phingou chatpa.
- *Agreement:* Proportion of sum of the true positive and true negative among the total number of women.
- *Kappa*: Agreement between observed and expected by chance.

3.7 LIMITATIONS OF THE STUDY

The present study was conducted to gather data on reproductive health of women in Manipur comparing two areas in Manipur. This comprehensive approach presents considerable methodological challenges which might compromise scientific rigor on the part of the study. Lack of resources forced to balance advantageous against disadvantageous of this approach. This study doesn't include men's perception of women's illnesses and their own sex related illnesses to fully understand men's role in transmission of infection to women as well as in influencing women's ability to report and seek care for reproductive morbidities.

4

Area and the People

4.1 A GLANCE AT INDIA AND MANIPUR

India is the second largest country in South Asia covering over three million squares kilometer from the Himalayas in the North to the Indian Ocean in the south. With a population of 1028.6 million (Census, 2001) it is the second most populous country in the world.Every year in India, roughly 30 million women experience pregnancy and 27 million have a live birth (MOHFW, 2003). Of these, over 100,000 maternal deaths occur annually.Maternal mortality rate, an important indicator of maternal health in India is estimated to be 407/100,000 live births (RGI, 1998). With an estimated 136,000 deaths, India has the highest burden of maternal mortality in the world.Direct evidence from NFHS suggests considerable rural and urban variation: the rural maternal mortality ratio was considerably higher than the urban in both the early and late 1990s; 434 as compared to 385 in NFHS-I, 619 and 267 respectively in NFHS-2. Thirty percent of ever-married women report at least one type of problem related to vaginal discharge. 18 percent reported symptom of urinary tract infection (UTI). Overall, 36 percent of women report either problems with vaginal discharge or symptom of UTI (NFHS-2) Sex ratio in India continues to be unfavorable to females with 933 females for every 1000 males (Census, 2001)

The socio-cultural determinant too has a cumulative effect on maternal health.A co-relation exists between the social inequality and maternal health.The female literacy rate in India is 54.3 percent (Census, 2001) and 21.6 percent of the total population in India are below the poverty line (CBHI, 2002). Poverty and illiteracy have a negative bearing on the maternal health.

A brief sketch on Manipur is warranted as this study was conducted in Manipur.Manipur is situated on a branch of the eastern Himalayas range which protrudes towards the south along the Indo-Myanmar border sketching between 93.03E and 94.78 E and latitude 23.80°N to 25.68°N. The total population in Manipur is 2,388,634 (Census, 2001). The overall sex ratio in Manipur is 978 females per 1000 (RGI, 2001). However, the rural sex ratio is comparatively lower with 938 per 1000 (RGI, 2001). The female literacy rate is 59.7 percent in comparison to the male literacy rate of 77.87 percent (RGI, 2001).

At the health front, symptoms of reproductive health problems were reported among 50.3 percent of women in urban areas, and 58.9 percent in rural areas of Manipur. The mainly reported symptoms of reproductive health are abnormal vaginal discharge (41.3 percent), urinary tract infection (29.5 percent), bad odour (17.5 percent) and bleeding during intercourse (NHHS-2). Among these women who reported symptoms of reproductive health problem, 73.6 percent do not seek any treatment. 10.7 percent go to an allopathic provider, 2.0 percent go to pharmacist, 0.6 percent to *maibi* (traditional birth attendant) (NHHS-2). This explicates the debilitating heath condition of women. However, the pictures in two areas with Manipur i.e. Andro a rural area and Kwakeithel, a peri urban needs to be unraveled.

4.2 Andro and Kwakeithel

Traversing through a narrow gorge towards the eastern part of Manipur sucking in the exquisite beauty of pine grouping sylvan surroundings and daunting hill slopes flaunted with pine-apple field lies this suburb, Andro. It is just 26 kilometers away from Imphal covering 2,994.03 acres. The total population in Andro is 8313 of which 4187 are male and 4126 are female. There are thirteen localities in Andro.

Kwakeithel lies in the Imphal west District of Manipur. For this study, I have taken up those areas in Kwakeithel which are included in the word No.10 of Municipal council.The total population of this ward is 7111. The total number of male is 3435 and female is 3676. This shows that the numbers of female exceeds the numbers of male in this area.

4.2.1 Family Types:

Family forms the backbone of social structure. As awhole,family is the unit of production as well as consumption. It acts as an educative unit and a socio-cultural agency. It secures as the primary unit of enculturation and socialization for an individual.Both in Andro and Kwakeithel the prevalence of nuclear household is high. 72 percent of the household in Andro are nuclear and 27.8 percent of household are joint while in Kwakeithel, 70.6 percent are nuclear and 29.4 percent of the household are joint.

4.2.2 Kinship:

In both Andro and Kwakeithel, household are patrilineal and patriarchal.Marriage is patrilocal. After marriage, a woman leaves her natal place and joins the family of the man she is married to.There, for the most of the early years of her marriage, she is under the control of her mother-in-law. Although the oldest male is the head of the joint family, the mother-in-law is said to hold the greatest power in the domestic sphere (Dubey and Edwards, 1986)

Ideally a young girl is socialized to be obedient, self sacrificing and contribute positively as wives and daughter-in-law in their new household after marriage.A girl is expected to spend more time in the immediate vicinity of the house assisting in the arduous domestic task, help to clean the house, fetch water; cook and act as nursemaids to the younger siblings. Besides the family and kinship, traditionally there are two main institutions which organize the society in Andro namely- *Loishang* and *Pana.*

4.2.3 *Pana:*

Pana is one of the most important institutions in Andro. The function of *pana* is to instill to the male members of Andro their mores and tradition, judicial, religious activities concerning the village. It also includes family matters within its propaganda. There is intricate relationship between *pana* system and the social life of Andro. One is functionless without the other. The social and cultural life of people in Andro has close and Ceaseless ties with the *pana* system. To be a complete Andro resident, one has to enroll in the *pana* system to get them acquainted with the social mores, customs and tradition of Andro.

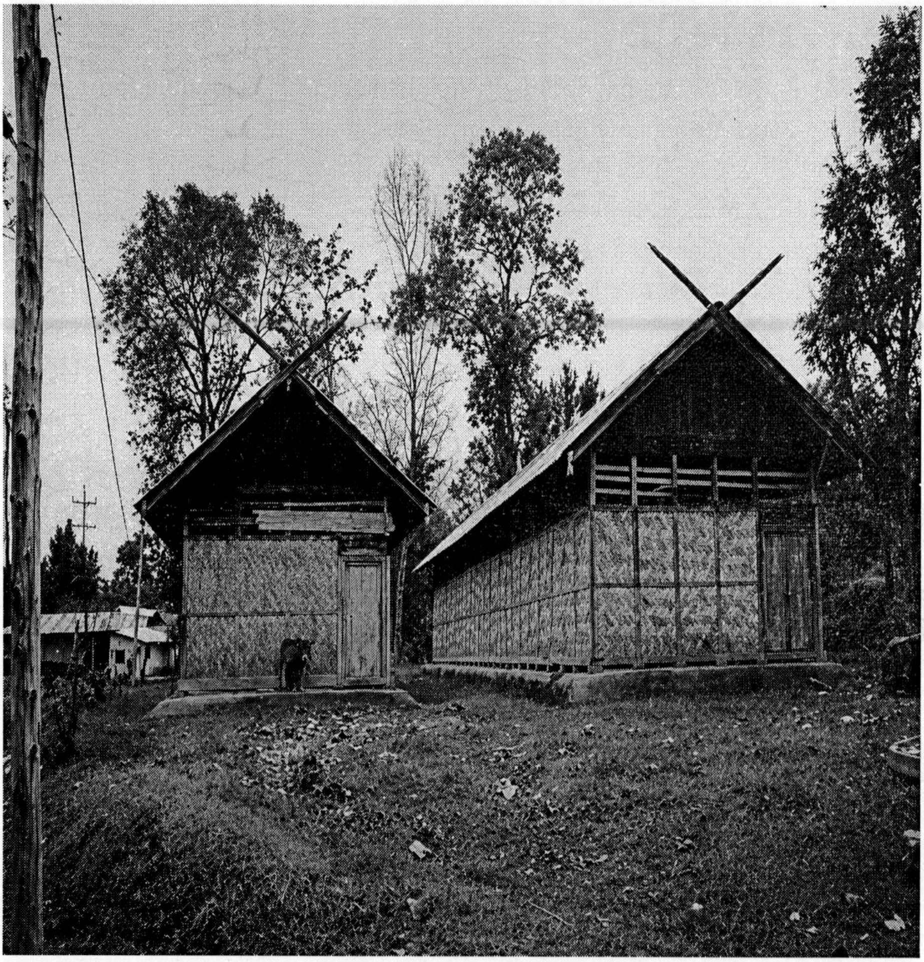

Figure 4.3: ***Pana in Andro***

4.2.4 *Loishang:*

Another important institution in Andro is *Loishang. Loishang* is the residing place of the deity *Panam ningthou* as well as the assembly hall where the chief of Andro and other nobleman carry out their administrative process interwined with religion. It acts as a judiciary court where all the seven nobleman takes decision conjointly with each other. The *Loishang* is thus a judiciary

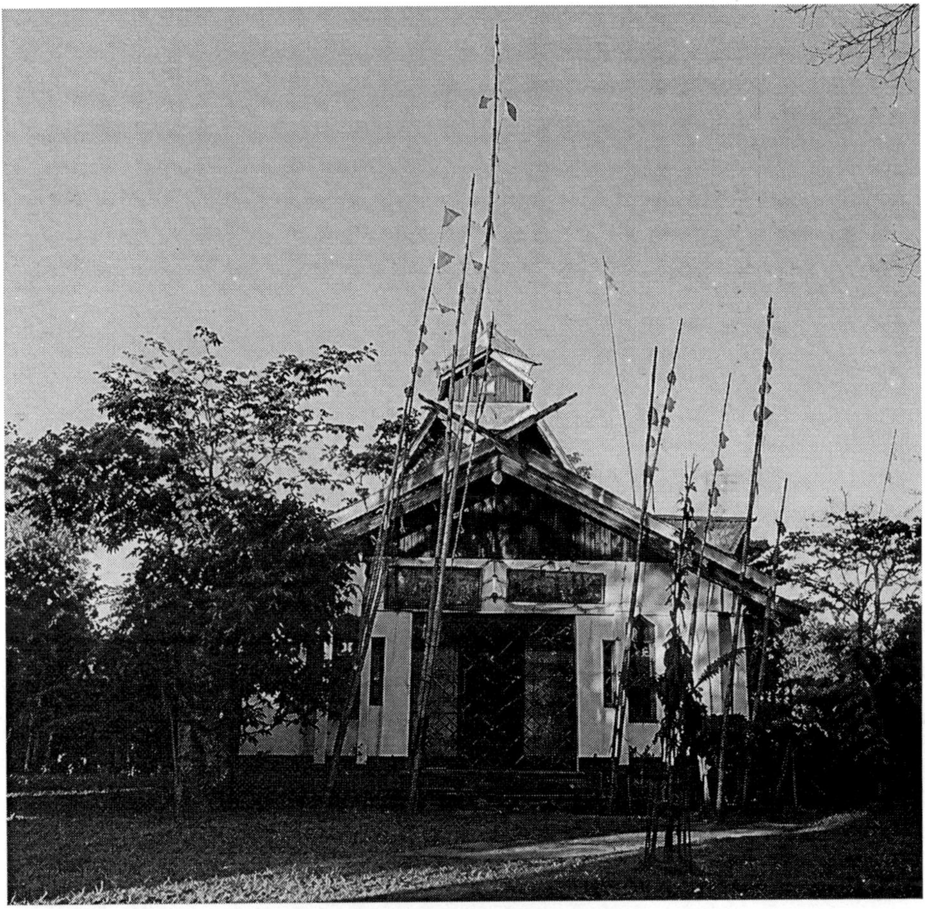

Figure 4.4: *Loishang* in Andro

Court-cum-temple which is considered as a sacred place. In the center of the *Loishang* there is a fireplace which is considered as sacred and cannot be extinguished. Thus, the *Loishang*is the rendezvous of judicial court with the platter of religious sacrament.

4.2.5 Religion:

Religion tends to be an important characteristic as it is often intertwined with mores and tradition. Andro society can be broadly classified into three different religious sections- one section consist of those who follows *Sanamahi*religion, another consist of those who have adopted Hinduism and the third section of those who have converted to Christianity. Sixty families having a population of three hundred approximately are found to have adopted Hinduism. Nearly 40 families comprising a population of about 200 people have accepted Christianity as their religion. The Christian society is divided into two groups following Baptism and Catholics. The Baptist group consists of nearly 170 members whereas 30 members were Catholic follower. Both the groups have established their separate mission school and church. The remaining majority are *Sanamahi* followers. In Andro, those members who convert themselves to Hindus or Christian keep a place separate for local household deity, *Lainingthou.*

In Kwakeithel, the main religion that they follow is Hinduism with sporadic *Sanamahi* and Christian followers.

4.2.6 Village Administration:

Village administration is carried out by the seven noblemen in Andro. Seven *Phamnaibai's* (noblemen) in Andro are: *Khullakpa, Luklakpa, Khunjahanba, Pakhanglakpa, Khabamlakpa, Yupanba and Naharakpa.* Each *Phamnaibai* is assigned with certain duties. They take decision in conjunction on certain issues arising within the village and those concerning their village and their decision are the most honored one. Their decision is vocalized by the *Khullakpa* (chief) and his word is final. Everybody bow before his decision. Any development program needs *Khullakpa's* permission before it is implemented in Andro society.

4.2.7 Association:

There are three main association found in Andro namely- all Andro youth club comprising of youths of the village, Mahila Mandal and *Meira Paibi* association.

All Andro youth club association is a voluntary organization.There are thirteen youth clubs in Andro.One, each in a leikai (locality) which is working under the supervision of All Andro youth club Association which was registered in 1977. They organize certain programmes like AIDS awareness programme, physical health training school, social camp, etc. They also encourage youths of the village in sports activities like football, handball, sepak takraw, etc. They provide free equipments and sports uniform.The club members work hand in hand with certain non-governmental organization in giving training for piggery farm.

Mahila Mandal Association which was founded in 1982, too has its role to play in development programmes implemented in Andro They give vocational training to women in tailoring, weaving, embroidery, etc. which helps women to earn a living of their own. At present, there are three Mahila Mandal Association- All Andro Mahila Mandal Association, Panthoibi Mahila Mandal Association and Khuman Mahila Mandal Association. Young girls are encouraged by these associations to participate in the field of sports. Besides these development programmes, a flavor of political activities are also added in their activities.Any issues concerning women are taken up by them.

The third association is the *Meira Paibi* Association.These are women's association. They are the torch bearer. They also function for the development of Andro society and also dissolve cases pertaining to women. The member's pool in money for funds and undertake development activities.It is a body through which women voice their grievances.

In Kwakeithel, the two associations which can take up developmental activities are the club and *Meira Paibi* association in each locality of Kwakeithel. These two bodies are strong in each locality of Kwakeithel.

4.2.8 Public Festivals:

Festivals are indispensable part of cultural life of the people in Andro and Kwakeithel. Every festival has legendary origin which acts as the governing factor in each of such gathering. Each season is marked by an appropriate festival in which ceremonies are related to warding off evil spirits or to bring peace and prosperity. Festivals are a medium of mass recreation. It is an occasion for feasting and rejoicing. There are common festivals which are celebrated both in Andro and Kwakeithel and there are some which are celebrated only in Andro like *lam haiba, kurak lamdaiba, khunthong lakpa, laisa tanba* and *saroi yenba, thasi lubak and laman chak pijaba.* Some of the festivals which are related with health are given below:

(i)Cheiraoba:

Cheiraoba is celebrated both in rural Andro and peri urban Kwakeithel. It is the New Year festival which takes place on the first day of the Meitei month *sajibu.* On this particular day, people clean their premises commerating the coming year. Deities, both inside and outside the residential premise are venerated and worshipped so as to appease them and guard them against any misfortune, disease and bless them for peace and prosperity in the forthcoming year. Delicious cuisines are prepared and offered to the deities for long life and prosperity of the members of the family.

(ii) Kurak Lamdaiba:

This festival is mainly performed to prevent cattle epidemic in Andro. This festival is performed mainly to shoo off evil spirits lurking around in the village in inaccessible parts like dense bush, river, stream, etc. beyond the village on the first Friday of August-September.

(iii) Khunthong Lakpa:

On the first Saturday of March a pig is sacrificed in *Panam Ningthou* temple. In the evening a white hen is offered. The offerings are made to the presiding deities of the four directions. The entry and outgoing people are halted when the ceremony is in process. All the shops in the market and roadside remain closed.

At the place where offerings are made a hole is dug out. After the ritual is over, the offerings are buried there. The neck of the hen is slashed and buried. This ceremony is to dispel off evil spirits beyond the community. The main objective of this ceremony is to appease evil spirits to protect against death and illness.

(iv) Laisa Tanba* and *Saroi Yenba:

For this festival, a male member from each household in Andro has to participate. The bachelor will hunt the animal. The hunted animal is hanged in front of the *Panam ningthou* temple. In the meantime, drums are beaten in a particular rhythm letting the whole community know that an animal is being hunted. After this the *sougrakpa* (nobleman who looks after the distribution of meat) will take down the animal, kill it and then skinned for meat. The person who hunted the animal will get the head of the animal. After cooking, the meat will be served to those present with local brew. The phenomenon behind this festival is to propitiate the deity to protect them from disease and illness.

(v) Lai Haraoba:

Lai haraoba is celebrated both in Andro and Kwakeithel. This festival is celebrated to appease the deities and seek blessing for peace prosperity and protect them from illness.

(vi) Saroi Khangba:

Saroi khangba is a ceremony which is performed to appease the evil spirits lurking around and free them from unnatural death and illness. This festival is celebrated in both Andro and Kwakeithel.

With the advent of Hinduism in Manipur, many festivals like Diwali, Durga Puja, etc. are also celebrated. In Andro, only Hinduised family celebrated these festivals.

4.2.9 Food and Drinks:

Food habit in Andro and Kwakeithel are almost same. However, consumption of meat is more in Andro than in Kwakeithel while the consumption of oil and spices is more in Kwakeithel. Rice is the staple food in both the areas. Fish is eaten and is the main ingredient in any dish in any form. Andro people lavish on long feast with hecatombs of fat cattle and oceans of spirituous drinks. In Kwakeithel, fish is main cuisine in feast. As in the verbose of Thaba, a woman of 23 years old, "We, Andro people eat, drink and rejoice to the hilth."

4.2.10 Dress and Ornaments:

People in Andro and Kwakeithel made a distinction of dress and ornaments that they flaunt depending on occasion and gender. For daily wear, men wear shirt with pant while for festive occasion they sport *dhoti* and *kurta*. For daily wear, women adorn with *phanek* and a blouse. These daily wear *phanek* are simple and plain. For festive occasion, the patterns of phanek are stripped one, the ground work of various colors. They complement with a blouse and a thin transparent *chaddar* with colorful design.

4.2.11 Language:

The Andro people speak *Meiteilon* dialect.However, there is intonational variation from the mainstream *Meiteilon* spoken by people in Kwakeithel.

It is believed that Andro *loi* belong to *chakpa loi,* a dialect different from the present dialect.However, but for a few words it is almost forgotten. Some linguist link the old dialect of Andro with the dialect spoken by the Sak tribe of Myanmar, F.K.Lehman, notable linguist established linguistic affinity of Andro of Manipur with that of the Sak tribe of Myanmar. Greison (1967) also wrote of the close connection of the old dialect of Andro with Kadu. Kadu is spoken in neighbouring Myanmar districts of Myitkyina, Katha and Upper Chindwin and Ganan. Ganan is merely a variant of Kadu and its speaker as well as those of Kadu called themselves as A-Sak. Thus, scholars link up the old dialect of Andro with Sak tribe.However, today, Andro loi are *Meiteilon* speakers though there is slight variation in tone and accent with the mainstream *Meiteilon* speakers including people from Kwakeithel.

4.2.12 Type and Distribution of House:

The dwelling house can be classified as traditional house which is kutcha with thatch roof, slightly modern which includes kutcha with tin roof and pucca with tin roof and modern house which is pucca house. In Andro, kutcha house with thatch roof are commonly found with 55.2 percent Kutcha/ pucca with tin roof at 41.2 percent and 36 percent of pucca house are found in Andro.

In Kwakeithel the traditional type of house are not found. 41.7 percent had kutcha house with tin roof 26.2 percent had pucca with tin roof and 32.1 percent had pucca house in Kwakeithel.

The houses in Andro are not sparely distributed. They tend to appear in cluster.Most of paddy field is adjacent to the residential area. The houses in Kwakeithel are densely distributed.There is congestion due to take of space.

4.2.13 Education:

One of the biggest disappointments with India's development has been education.Education can be a great lever to make a difference and an en route for successful addressal of health related issues.

There are 21 schools in Andro, among them, twelve are primary schools and nine are high schools. In Andro, as a non formal educational system- Anganwadi and Adult education are found.The adult education policy was active in the initial stage i.e. around 1990s but later as the old women/ adult were exhausted after the hectic circadian activities they could not attend the classes regularly.Thus everything comes to a stand still now.

There was a significant difference in the literacy level between males and females in Andro.46.9 percent of females and 73.2 percent of male were literate and 53.1 percent of females and 26.8 percent of males were illiterate.

The literacy rate of women in Kwakeithel was comparatively high with 79.1 percent though lesser than males which was 96.4 percent, 20.9 percent of females and 5.6 percent of male were illiterate.

Thus it can be surmise that literacy level was higher in Kwakeithel than in Andro.Moreover, the females in Kwakeithel have high percentage of literacy than females in Andro.

4.2.14 Occupation:

In Andro, due to low literacy level in the population most of the males and females were engaged in unskilled jobs. 68.5 percent of male, were cultivators.In Andro, agriculture is their mainstay.It is a family enterprise. Besides agriculture, there are some lucrative jobs which form their main occupation like weaving, brewing brew, pottery, basket making reed mat making, etc. Pottery, weaving and brewing brew are women's domain while basket making, reed mat making are done by man though there is no taboo attached to woman pursuing such kind of activities, 23.0 percent of women were engaged in pot making, 40.0 percent in weaving and 36.6 percent in brewing brewin Andro. In Kwakeithel, 15.0 percent of women were working as government employees.Only 1.6 percent of women were engaged in weaving. A good number of women (64.7 percent) are housewives.Comparatively males (41.7 percent) were employed more in government offices, 25 percent were engaged in business and 33.2 percent were engaged as rickshaw pullers, drivers, petty shop owners, etc.

4.2.15 Economy:

In Andro, majority of the household had family income Rs 1000-4000 per month. The mean family income in Andro was Rs 3972.50.In Kwakeithel, the family income ranging from Rs 5000-9000 was highest with 32.6 percent. The mean family income was Rs 11,925.

Table 4.1: Frequency of Type of House, Type of Family and Income in Andro and Kwakeithel.

CHARACTERISTICS	ANDRO (N=200) (%)	KWAKEITHEL (N=200) (%)
Type of Houses		
Kutcha house with thatch roof	55.2	0
Kutcha house with tin roof.	39.7	41.7
Pucca house with tin roof	1.5	26.2
Pucca house	3.6	32.1
Type of Family		
Nuclear	72.2	70.6
Joint	27.8	29.4
Income		
1000-4000	78.4	25.7
5000-9000	16.5	32.6
10,000-14000	3.6	15.5
15000-19000	0	8.0
20,000-24000	1.5	8.6
25,000-29,000	0	4.8
30,000-34,000	0	3.7
35,000-39,000	0	0
40,000-44,000	0	0
45,000-49,000	0	0
50,000-54,000	0	1.5

4.2.16 Ventilation:

The knowledge about ventilation is measured by the number of room, doors and windows that a house has.In Andro the mean number of room was 3.54, door was 2.99 and the mean number of windows was 3.15.

In Kwakeithel, the mean number of door, windows and room were higher.The mean number of room was 5.27, door was 5.28 and a window was 6.67, which shows that people in Kwakeithel that better knowledge about ventilation.

4.2.17 Sanitation and Hygiene:

(i) Source of Water:

The source of water is one of the indicators of sanitation and hygiene. If there is scarcity of water then women will have to bear the brunt of fetching the water and in maintaining a clean surrounding in their vicinity and in maintaining personal hygiene. In Andro, the main source of water for cleaning and washing are pond and stream water. However, for drinking and cooking purpose, the main sources of water are spring water, hand-pump and tap water.23.5 percent use tap water, 27.5 percent use hand pump and 49.0 percent use spring water in Andro as potable water.

In Kwakeithel, the source of water for washing and cleaning are pond and tap water.For drinking and cooking purpose they use only tap water.

(ii) Place and Material used for Cooking:

The place of cooking and the material used for cooking will explicate the hygienic practices of people in Andro and Kwakeithel. In Andro, 11.5 percent of household cook inside the hutment in common space, 6.5 percent cook outside the hutment in a separate kitchen and 82.0 percent use to cook inside the hutment in a separate room. Firewood is the most commonly used fuel with 80.0 percent. 19.0 percent of the household employed Liquified Petroleum Gas as fuel and 0.5 percent use kerosene stove. Countable number of houses had hand made chimney.

Table 4.2:
Frequency of the Source of Water, Place for Cooking, Fuel for Cooking, Place for Throwing Garbage, Place for Throwing Animal Waste

CHARACTERISTICS	ANDRO (N=200) (%)	KWAKEITHEL (N=200) (%)
Source of drinking water		
Tap water	23.5	100
Hand pump	27.5	0
Spring water	49.0	0

CHARACTERISTICS	ANDRO (N=200) (%)	KWAKEITHEL (N=200) (%)
Place for cooking		
Inside the hutment in common space	11.5	0
Outside the hutment in a separate kitchen	6.5	10.0
Inside the hutment in a separate kitchen	82.0	90.0
Fuel for cooking		
Firewood	80.0	1.5
LPG	19.0	97.0
Kerosene stove	0.5	1.5
Place for Throwing Garbage		
Open	58.5	1.5
Pit hole	35.5	84.0
Drainage	6.0	14.5
Place for Throwing Animal Waste		
Pit hole	42.0	2.5
Open	34.5	1.0
Both	0.5	9.5
No Cattle	23.0	87.0

The households in Kwakeithel cook outside the hutment in a separate kitchen (10.0 percent) while 90.0 percent cook inside the hutment in a separate kitchen.The most frequently utilized fuel in Kwakeithel was Liquified Petroleum Gas with 97.0 percent and minimal number of household use firewood (1.5 percent) and stove (1.5 percent).

(iii) Place for Throwing Garbage:

The place for throwing waste has an important role in adumbrating the sanitation and hygiene of an area.In Andro there are three ways of throwing the garbage throw it in the open, throw it in drainage and drying a pithole to dump the wastage.A large number of households throw garbage in open (58.5 percent), 35.5 percent throw in a pithole and 6.0 percent throw the wastage in the drainage.

In Kwakeithel, 84.0 percent throw the garbage in the pithole, 14.5

percent in the drainage and 1.5 percent in the open. The behaviour of throwing waste in the drainage and in the open shows that there is lack of knowledge about sanitation and hygiene.

The management of animal waste is also another criterion for maintenance of sanitation. In Andro, 42.0 percent throws the waste in a pit hole, 34.5 percent throw in the open and 0.5 percent throws the waste in both ways.

In Kwakeithel, 87.0 percent of household doesn't have cattle. 2.5 percent of the remaining of household throw the animal waste in pithole, 1.0 percent in open and 9.5 percent throw the waste in both ways.

(iv) Toilet:

Having proper toilet facility is essential for healthy existence.There are four type of toilet- open, where people ease off in the field behind a bush or in any piece of land, pit hole, where a hole is dug up and covered on all the four directions with rags, tin sheets or wooden plank with tin roof. Semi pucca has more or less the same structure but the floor is cemented and pucca where the structure are made up of concrete.

In Andro, 81.0 percent do not have toilet facility. 10.5 percent used semi-pucca, 5.05 use pucca and 3.5 percent use pithole whereas in Kwakeithel none of the household shat in the open, 0.5 percent used pit hole, 70.0 percent used semi pucca and 29.5 percent use pucca toilet.

4.2.18 Transport and Communication:

One of the main factors in health issues is transport and communication. Distance limits women's access to health care particularly when appropriate transportation is in limited supply and communication difficult. In Andro, the roads are dusty in sunny days and muddy on rainy days. One gets lost in cloud of dust when any vehicles pass by. On rainy days the shoe gets stuck in the mud. However, it was refreshing to walk down the road and lanes in Andro. Within Andro, people commute in two wheelers like scooter but bicycle is the most common way to glide along. Covering distance by foot is also a common sight in Andro. 1.5 percent had car, 6.0 percent had scooter and 30.0 percent had cycle in Andro.

If one has to go beyond Andro then buses and jeep are the main means of commuting though some use their own vehicles like scooter or car. However, the frequency is very less. To reach the hospital, which is in Imphal, they have to wait for the bus at the main route of Andro, which will drop them at one area of Imphal. From this area they have to traverse either by rickshaw, scooter or jeep to reach the hospital.

For commuting from one place to another or to the hospital there are varieties of means of transportation in Kwakeithel. They can easily access the health care. Buses, jeep and rickshaw ply in every nook and corner of the road. Moreover, they have their own vehicles too. 49.5 percent own scooter, 62.5 percent had bicycle and 32.7 percent had car.

4.2.19 Market Place:

In Andro, there is one main market where only woman sells vegetables, fish, banana, etc. There are few petty shops in Andro with minimal stock supply of basic grocery provision such as sugar, onion, salt, pulses, etc. Women from the neighbouring villages come and sell their things. Besides these shops and women vendor there were few hotels also which sell local brew, pork, beef, etc.

In Kwakeithel, there is a main market commonly known as Kwakeithel bazaar where people from hills and villages bring their commodities and sell. Most of daily requirements are available in Kwakeithel bazaar.The shops are mostly run by male though females are also seen running the shops. However, the vegetables and fruit lane are women's domain. Male members are not allowed to transgress as vendor but can enter as buyers.

4.2.20 Health Care Facilities:

In Andro, there is one primary health centre where there is one doctor, two nurses, two-health supervisors, three-health workers, one laboratory technician and one microscopist. The main activities carried out in Primary Health Centre are routine curative care, tuberculosis detection, maternal and child health services such as diarrhea disease control, immunization and family planning.

There are two pharmacy shops in Andro which are run by layman with stock of common medicine for cold, cough, diarrhea, vitamin tablets, etc.

People in Kwakeithel can get access to a variety of medical facilities.

Many clinics and hospitals are available within their reach. The availability and accessibility of the health care facility is one of the important factors in the domain of health.

5

Women's Perception of Body

All systems of knowledge are socially constructed. Folk biology, however, has an exceptional resilience and power over people's behavior and understandings since it does not seem to be socially constructed to local participants (Jeffery et al., 1988). This chapter attempts to explore how women perceive different organs of their body, their location, interrelationships of different parts of the body and their functioning. It is an endeavour to present their beliefs about their body (ethno-anatomy) and body functions (ethno-physiology) and the different practices which they follow in accordance with these beliefs. It is based on locally perceived processes that affect women's reproductive health status and describes those beliefs and practices about women's bodies that emerged as the most important in the context of women's illnesses.

Information presented in this chapter has been collated from data collected in the ethnographic phase. Information regarding childbirth, pregnancy rites, delivery and post partum practices, family planning methods, etc. was also procured. Besides, observation and focus group discussion with the traditional birth attendants and the ordinary village women help to sketch out the graphic representation of the ethno-anatomical and ethno-physiological models. For this body-mapping was used. On probing and questioning, women were able to give better insights of their bodies and describe them in detail. The figures drawn by typical village women and traditional birth attendants serve as a guide to the discussion of findings of ethno-anatomy and ethno-physiology in their socio-cultural context. It was found that traditional birth attendants were more aware of the physiological processes than an ordinary woman.

5.1 ONSET AND LEARNING ABOUT MENSTRUATION

Menarche symbolized the attainment of physical maturity and ability to bear children. *Thagi khongkap lakpa* (coming of monthly period) or *mangba* (polluted) were the local terms used for menstruation and were justified by its occurrence once a month and segregation of women during this period. Flowery terms like *lei lakpa* (coming of flower) are also used as metaphor for menstruation. Menstruation is used allegorical to the blooming of flower.

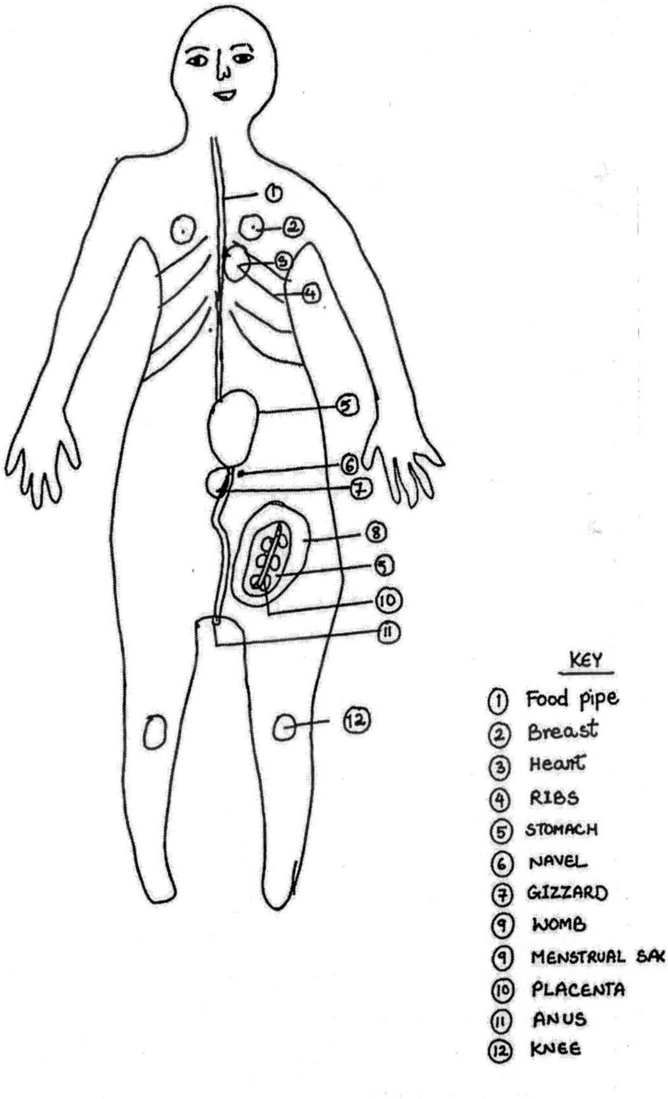

Figure 5.1: Body Map (Village Women)

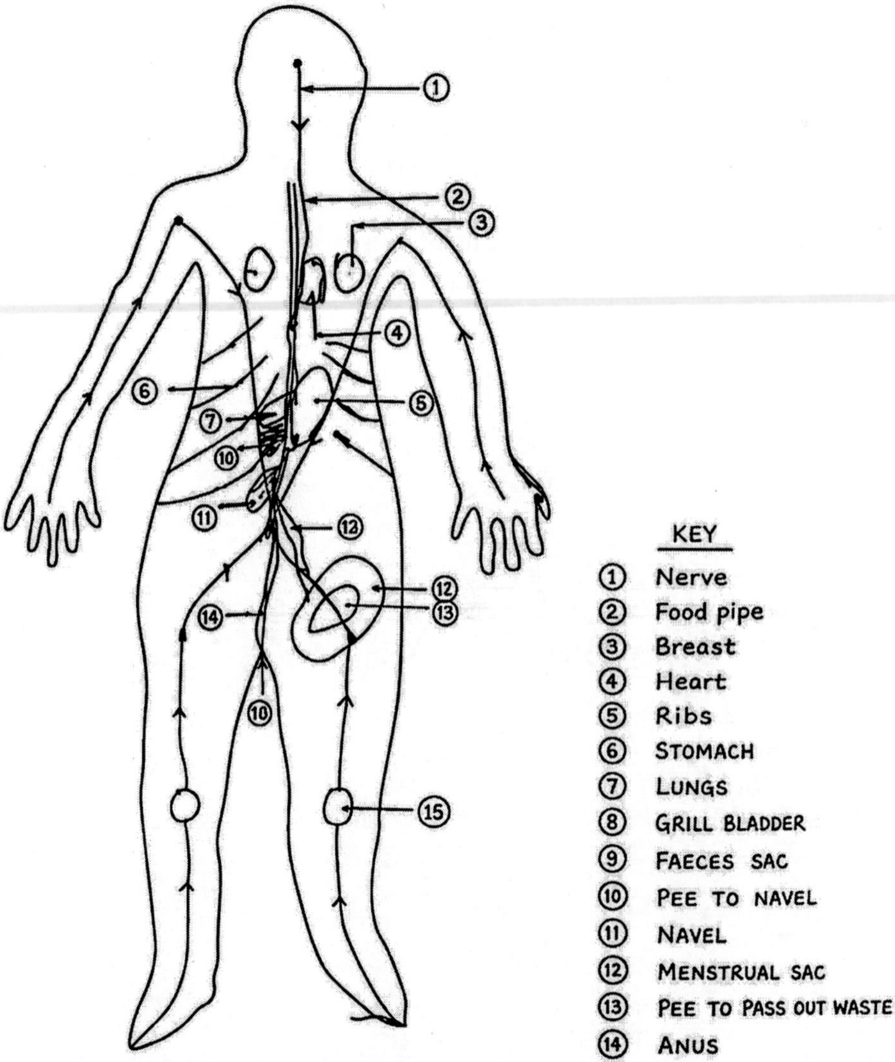

Figure 5.2: Body Map (Traditional Birth Attendant)

In the verbose of Hemsori, a *maibi* in Andro:

"Menstrual blood comes out from a lotus shaped sac which is located inside the womb where the baby stays. It blooms once in a month. Every month when it blooms blood comes out".

Most of the young girls reportedly knew about menstruation before their marriage from different sources. A young girl evolves into a stage of an unmarried maiden locally termed as *leisabi* (who moves like a flower) with the onset of menstruation. In Andro, with this status they are allowed to perform dance in one of their biggest festival, *lai haraoba.* Becoming a *leisabi* is publicly declared. The *pakholoi* (messenger) from *Koso* (dormitory) will inform of their *leisabi* status. They register their name in *Koso* (dormitory) during *lai haraoba* festival. The *leisabi* status ensures them of their participation in *lai haraoba* festival.

To bring light to the situation Thoibi, 37 years old woman in Andro recalls:

> "When I reach sixteen years, I was informed of my *leisabi* status. I was ecstatic when I perform dance in the *lai haraoba* festival. My name was publicly declared and was given the service of taking care of *Panam Ningthou* ".

> Thaba, a young *leisabi* of 22 years old in Andro who was weaving a woolen *phanek* on a loom responded:

> "I was too embarrassed to tell my mother and sister when my first menstruation started. So, I didn't tell them but my mother came to know about it as my clothes got soiled. Then, my mother asked me whether I have started with my periods. I gave a positive reply and she showed me how to wear *phanek* during menstruation."

> Santa, a 20 years old *leisabi* in Kwakeithel recalls:

> "My menstruation started when I was at school. I was shocked and surprised at the same time. I came home and told my mother about it."

Menstruation is therefore a public affair in Andro.Mothers, sisters, friends or neighbouring women orient her in the process of menstruation. Once a girl attains a *leisabi* status certain restrictions are imposed on her so as to keep her reminding of her reproductive power which should be contained till marriage. So, during the liminal period between menarche and marriage she is carefully guarded by her natal or patrilineal male kins. As the cliché goes "whether a petal falls on a thorn or a thorn falls on a petal, it is the petal which is hurt", here petal is coterminous with unmarried women and thorn with male. This drives home the delicacy and onus of boundary maintenance by a women after she attain the status of a *leisabi*.

5.1.1 Menstrual Pad and Menstrual Practices:

In Andro, most of the girls do not wear panties, when they are at home. On the contrary, women feel uncomfortable staying without wearing panties in Kwakeithel. In Andro, the main reason for not wearing panties during menstruation is that it will obstruct the flow of bad blood coming out. They consider that blood coming out during menstruation is bad blood. If all the bad blood is not taken out then one will become ill and the body will become weak. This belief also prevails among women in Kwakeithel. However, in their quest to adjust with modern lifestyle they adopted the practice of wearing panties.

Tamu, one *maibi* in Andro responded:

> "Now-a-days people have started wearing panties that's why they have become weak and their complexion is not glowing. How can they look beautiful and remain healthy when they do not let the bad blood come out of the body."

In Kwakeithel, women wear disposable sanitary pad or clothes which are folded and stitched on the panties. However, women in Andro wear two to three *phanek,* one on top of the other. They will wear the innermost *phanek* like a dhoti, pulling up one end and tucking in on the back side. When they are at home or visit their neighbours they do not wear panties. Only when they go out of village they wear panties with clothes folded and sewn on the panties. 25.3 percent of women in Andro use *phanek* while 74.7 percent of women use clothes when they go out of the village or to the neighbouring localities. In Kwakeithel, when women stay inside the house, 23.2 percent wear *phanek,* 43.7 percent use cloth and 32.2 percent use sanitary napkin. When women go out, 44.7 percent use cloths, 55.3 percent use sanitary napkin.

Thus this accounts that women in Andro prefer to use *phanek* when they are at home without any undergarments as it is believed that wearing panties will block the flow of the menstrual blood which is considered as bad. Women perceive that if this bad blood remains inside the body then one's health will deteriorate. Women in Andro did not use sanitary napkin. The most commonly used material when a woman goes out is a piece of cloth folded sewn inside the panties. The material can be either an old piece of *phanek* or an old piece of cloth. However in Kwakeithel, women prefer wearing undergarment when they go outside their house. They have also started using sanitary napkin as menstrual pad.

The *phanek* and clothes are washed with soap in cold water. Some use Dettol while washing in Kwakeithel. Before discarding clothes they will wash the blood properly as it is believed that if they throw clothes with menstrual blood, the women will become weak and her health will deteriorate. The washed clothes are often not dried in open. They consider it improper in front of male members to spread out *phanek*/clothes in the open. So, they try to hide it beneath some clothes.

One interesting menstrual practices which women in this area observe is related to the pollution aspect of menstrual blood; a concept which is prevalent across many states in India (Jeffery and Jeffery, 1989; Nichter, 1989). Women are considered polluted during menstruation. People believe that menstrual blood is bad thus, is considered as polluted. Traditionally, a menstruating woman was confined inside a room. However, in today's generation, they are not confined but still are considered polluted and are prohibited from preparing food and entering the culturally defined area of Gods and Goddesses. Certain granaries may not be entered by menstruating women. This situation is relaxed in Kwakeithel. Women wait 5-7 days after the first day of their menstruation to take bath which is when their menstrual period is getting over. Euphemistically, it is "washing their hair" on the 5th or 7th day of a menstrual period. The numbers of days vary according to the number of days for each woman's menstrual period. The reasoning behind this practice is to cleanse oneself of the "polluting" menstrual blood. The bed linen, pillow cover, mosquito net is supposed to be washed on the day when they take bath after their menstruation period.

During menstruation women are not allowed to have sex and it is considered bad for both men and women. There is a belief that men will become henpecked if they have sex when a women is menstruating and that for the women who is menstruating, she will become weak. Thus, avoidance of sexual intercourse is practiced during menstruation.

Some of the symptoms women had before menstruation are the craving to have sour things, *puk naba* (pain in the abdomen), *ethan thangatpa* (feeling bloated up), *khwang naba* (back pain).

5.2 SEXUAL FUNCTION

People use a variety of euphemisms when talking about sexual intercourse. Coy terms like man and woman meeting, doing things, being together or sleeping on the same bed are used to represent sexual intercourse. Sexual interactions are generally initiated by men. Although women's sexual desires are not explicitly spoken of, an older woman explained the following:

> "When women show more flesh and wears tight clothes to attract the attention of man, which man can resist? Both man and woman are equal partners and have desires."

Sexual encounter between husband and wife are accepted as norm. Women do speak disapprovingly of "other" sexual encounter. If young unmarried woman had sexual relationship with a man and get pregnant then, the boy who makes her pregnant has to marry her. Even if the girl is not pregnant but if they are caught in an uncompromising position the boy has to marry the girl or woman. If the sexual encounter is without the consent of the girl or women then certain actions are taken up by the village head (*khullakpa*) in Andro.

Women also spoke about abstinence from sex at certain times. There is a strong belief that it is impure to have intercourse during menstruation. Similarly, sexual intercourse soon after childbirth is unadvisable. During post partum period women are considered to be in a tender conditions and weak. They are considered as impure for a period of four month after childbirth. Their blood is considered as tender (*e-nouba*) thus, sexual abstinence is practiced. It is believed that if a couple violates the practice it would adversely affect the women's health and will lead to such an illness known as *nupa mangba* (male polluted). In such a condition, the woman lacks appetite and starts puking, even at the sight of food. Her whole body will shrink and finally she will die. They believe that even doctor cannot cure such ailment except the *maiba* (traditional healer).

One woman elucidates:

> "My son-in-law is a sex maniac. My daughter gave birth to a daughter last year. Before four months she had this illness (*nupa mangba*). Luckily, the *maiba* (traditional healer) gave her medicines and thus saved her

otherwise she would have just passed away. We saved her just in the nick of time".

Sexual abstinence is strictly practiced during peurperium. Non-observance is reprimanded by household elders and other close relatives. The above findings implicates that sexual abstinence is strictly followed during menstruation and peurperium.

5.3 CONCEPTION

Cessation of menstruation to a woman marks her pregnancy. Additionally the retention of blood is evidenced in symptoms such as nausea, vomiting and rashes. According to *maibi* in Andro the women's blood which comes out during menstruation and male's *mahik* (germ) come together to form a child. However, according to village women there are many placentas inside the womb of a woman. The male *mahik* (germ) will enter inside the placenta and form a child. If the germ enters on the right side then one will give birth to a male child and if it enters on the left side it will give birth to a female child.

In the verbose of one *maibi* in Andro:

"Man's *mahik* (germ) enters the woman's body and go to the womb where it meets the woman's blood and baby is formed."

In Andro, women rarely consult a *maibi* or nurse or doctor when pregnancy starts. They rely on their own diagnosis. In Kwakeithel women generally go to a doctor to consult and confirm about their status once menstruation stops. All women note the start of their menstruation according to a lunar calendar and if their next period does not begin they consider that one month is completed. Once pregnancy is confirmed then the women is not allowed to do any hard labor but pregnancy is also not seen as an occasion for rest.

As one woman put it:

"Movement and working is healthy for a pregnant woman and will help her in delivering the baby with less pain".

Women consider that pregnancy should last between nine and ten lunar months. Women believe that if the baby is born prematurely in the even months i.e. 6th and 8th month of pregnancy then the baby will die but if it is born on 7th and 9th month of pregnancy then the baby will live.

The maibi accounts:

In the first month of pregnancy, it is just a clot of blood without any eyes or nose or any defined body parts. Life enters the baby only on the third month. Then, its body parts begin to develop. Female foetuses moves earlier than the male, a male baby are lodged on the woman's right side while a female baby reside on the left side. By about seven months, the baby is fully formed but spends the rest of the pregnancy growing and gaining strength drinking blood and water inside the womb. The developing foetus takes its strength from the mother's retained menstrual blood.

5.3.1 Pregnancy Rites:

During this stage, a woman along with the physiological change has to abide certain restrictions imposed on her in terms of food habit and movement. A pregnant woman is abstained from any social as well as household religious ceremonies. Pregnancy, the creation of life must not be brought into contact with death. Hence, the pregnant woman as well as the father of the child should not participate in mortuary or funeral rites. At this stage, she and her husband cannot kill any living creature or certain mystically dangerous animal else his wife may miscarry or bear an abnormal or deformed child. A pregnant woman is restricted from walking in the dark, in the hot afternoons and eating in the market as she could invite spirits lurking in those places to follow her and harm the baby.

5.4 *ANGANG POKPA* (CHILDBIRTH)

Childbirth is a universal human experience. However, the birth experience takes place in a cultural context and is shaped by the views and practices of that culture.This section will discuss the childbirth process with reference to the following issues: *Maibi,* the childbirth attendant,the childbirth and the post partum period.

5.4.1 Child birth Attendant (*Maibi*):

In Andro, most of the deliveries were conducted by *maibi*, the traditional birth attendant or by more knowledgeable older women of the household in the absence of *maibi.* By feeling the pulse beat of the pregnant woman, a maibi can predict the timing of childbirth. Women consider that pregnancy ends in the tenth lunar month. So, once the pregnant woman reaches the tenth month the family members are alert and started taking care for the day. They called the *Maibi* frequently to check the pulse beat. In Andro, there is no separate place for childbirth. Two weeks ahead of the predicted date of delivery preparations started. Two bundles of straw which are of good quality are spread out in the sun and old phanek are washed and kept for use.

Women make clear distinction between *Maibi* and other experienced women who help in delivering babies. *Maibi's* are considered polluted and expect some form of payment in return for their service. The payment may be in the form of money, food stuffs etc. Most of the *maibi's* in Andro are old widows. People do not eat the food cooked by the *maibi's*. Even if she has husband and family once she becomes a *maibi* she has to live and eat separately as they are considered *mangba* (polluted). A *maibi* will wash the child and mother as well as the soiled clothes after cutting the umbilical cord. Other women who help in conducting delivery will leave once the child is given birth. Cleaning of the mother and child will be done by the *maibi* with the help of family members. The umbilical cord is cut only by the maibi. Cutting of umbilical cord is considered defiling so, any woman who conducts the delivery cuts the umbilical cord then they also becomes a *maibi* and thus considered as polluted. However, if the umbilical cord is cut by a male he does not become a *maibi* and so, is not considered as polluted. He can purify himself after taking bath. So, for a woman, once defiled is always defiled.

Hemsori, a maibi in Andro talks about her services.

> "Nobody taught me. I learned everything by myself. I watched and learned from my own body. No mishaps happen in all my deliveries".

As a *maibi* she goes to any household that calls her and does all the work which is associated with delivery. As a result, she expects payment for her services. Primarily, deliveries are almost exclusively a woman's domain including household women; *maibi's* and sometimes nurse from the primary health center. However, if the *maibi*, nurse or doctor in primary health center warns of any complication they go to hospitals in Imphal for delivery as there is inadequate infrastructure for any complication in delivery.

Maibi's fully understand the importance of recognizing complications.

Abnormal presentation protracts labor, endangering both mother and child so, *maibi* tries to asses if the baby is straight and correctly positioned i.e. with the head engaging on the cervix, inverted i.e. a footling breech or askew or obstructed i.e. transverse some *maibi's* claim of the caliber to turn a baby even during labor. Others said that it is difficult during late pregnancy but they can lay their hand in case of a footling breech presentation though not a transverse one. They have no foetal trumpets or other means of detecting foetal distress except feeling the women's belly. The *maibi's* themselves said that they cannot remedy problem like failure of cervical dilation, transverse lie, cords entangled on the neck of the baby, over-long pregnancy. So, if a maibi diagnose a problem she is likely to withdraw from the case. They generally claimed that they had never had serious mishaps for that very reason.

> "I examine the woman first and judge if she and the baby are all right. If there is any complication, I told them that it is beyond my competence and cannot handle the case". (Maibi)

> "In difficult cases, I refuse to put my hand on the women. I send them to big hospitals in Imphal". (Maibi)

5.4.2 An Account of Childbirth:

This section describes the actual childbirth process as observed once and also present findings from women's report in the ethnographic phase. A pregnant woman will continue her normal daily domestic chores until the moment she feels contractions. The room where she stays is usually the place where she gives birth which is generally away from the men and children of the household. The sun dried straws are spread out on the floor and on top of which the phanek are spread out. A hole is dug up at the corner of the room where she will give birth and stay after giving birth to throw the waste and blood. While giving birth, not only the *maibi,* but also some elderly women and young women are required to help the maibi and the woman who is going to deliver the baby. Once when the contraction starts the pregnant women is sanctified with smokes of cultic herbs called *khoichum-leikham* to dispel off evil spirits. The women in labor pain will squat and a healthy woman will sit in front to support her sitting on a bagful of rice or on a high stool. She will clutch the woman when she frets and moves to bear the labor pain. She is called as *maiyoknabi* (the one who face). Another woman will light up the hand made bamboo torch and there was no current and proper ventilation. In one corner of the room is a little fire place which is continually stokėd by a woman to heat the materials required during the delivery. All the women of the household usually participate in the process, some of whom are more active than the others. An older, grandmotherly woman who is more experienced will supervise the women who are assisting the delivery process.

In her absence the next senior most women will take charge. The older woman will sit and instruct the younger ones to make tea for the woman in labor and for the woman who are attending the birth. The woman who is going to deliver in also fed with local brew which they believe will enhance the delivery process. As the contraction continues, the attending woman tries to check the position of the child to assess the case.

Hemsori Explains:

"The most difficult delivery is when the baby is in transverse position. When labor pain starts I try to straighten the child from outside by massaging the stomach with my hand and then insert my finger inside the woman's vagina to check if I can feel the child's head."

Women who are assisting the *maibi* will help in massaging the laboring women's stomach gently on the side; feed her with hot pork/chicken soup or tea. Every now and then the *maibi* will wash her finger and insert again into the woman's vagina to check how far up she can feel the infant's head.

If the depth is till the wrist it means that it will take 1½ hour. However, if it is till the finger length then only half an hour is left. Thereby, the *maibi* can tell the how long will the labor take. When she takes out her finger she wipes them on the *phanek* which is spread out occasionally dipping in water to clean them.

The normal labor time is one day. However, if it exceeds more than a day then women consider it as a problem and resort to nurse or taking the women to the hospital. Although a long labor is considered a problem it is considered normal to experience pain during labor and a woman is not encouraged to become hysterical or cry out loudly during the delivery.

Hemsori retorts:

"Shut up. Don't you think about the consequence when you have pleasure?"

"When you can't bear this pain why do you want to have sex" another woman rebukes.

Some women who experience labor pain learn to bear it by calling out her mother and ancestor and holding onto the woman who attend the childbirth. Some bear it by hurting oneself.

One woman exclaims:

"When I gave birth to my first child I bit my lower lip so hard to bear the labor pain that blood started coming out".

As the labor pain continues women continue to give hot soup and shake her stomach around. She is encouraged to sit up and squat. Eventually when the amniotic fluid sac burst the attending women believe that the child is on the way. As the head of the infant starts emerging all the attending women starts urging the laboring mother to push harder and harder. As soon as the infants head emerge out of the vagina the *maibi* pulls out the rests of the body which follows through very quickly. The *maibi* pummels the stomach, so that the *naopham* (placenta) will come out.

There are times when the placenta does not come out. In such cases, the maibi will throw out a *kangkhil maru* out of the house through a hole which the maibi made on the wall where *Lainingthou* (household deity) stays. If the placenta still doesn't come out then the family members will call the *maiba* (traditional healer) to make offering to God.

When the *naopham* (placenta) comes out the maibi will cut the umbilical cord either with a new blade / *toubak or wakthou.* The belief of cutting the umbilical cord with *wakthou* is that the child will grow tall and sturdy like a *wakthou* bamboo.

5.5 POST PARTUM BELIEFS AND PRACTICES

After cutting the umbilical cord the *maibi* will bathe the baby in lukewarm water. After circumambulating the fire, the baby is wrapped by clean piece of cloth which is passed through fire so as to dispel off evil spirits and then the baby is kept on the left side of mother. The phanek which is soiled during childbirth is taken out and covered with new piece of cloth. The sleeping place of the mother is made separately. The bed is made out of straw and is near the fireplace. For three months she has to sleep on this bed. For few days urination, defecation is done inside the house. For three days the baby will be fed by neighbouring breastfeeding mother. The mother will start breastfeeding the baby after three days.

After cutting the umbilical cord and bathing the baby, the placenta will be taken up in *khangra* leaf. 'If it is a baby boy then the placenta is wrapped in five layers of *khangra* leaf and then screwed up with five stripes of cane. It is then placed inside a small earthen pot. In case of girl child the placenta is wrapped in six layers of *khangra* leaf screwed up with six stripes of cane. Then, the earthen pet containing placenta is sanctified with smokes of cultic herbs called *khoichum-leikham* to dispel off evil spirit and then buried at a depth of about two inch inside the house near the main door. If the baby is male, the pot is burned on the right side. In case of female child it is buried on the left side by the father. They believe that if they bury the placenta inside the house then, the person die in an unknown place of unknown illness.

On the third day after giving birth, purificatory rite is performed by *maibi*. For this, water from *eshaiphu* is taken in a pitcher and then sprinkled in and around the house and to all the members of the family with a leafy branch of *tairen* and *pungphai*. Until and unless this purification rite is performed granary of the house is not allowed to open and members of the lineage are abstained from attending any religious or public festivals as they are considered polluted. If this purificatory rite is performed all are purified except the new mother. The new mother will be considered polluted for three months. The place where she stays should be near a fireplace. Everyday fire is stoked. They believe that fire has medicinal value. It heals the woman faster and helps in removing out the *e-manai* (remnant blood and pus inside the womb) thereby making the woman recuperates faster. They also apply *yu machin* (local brew) which enhance in the process of healing. During this confinement period, women also practice *khwangehet punba* abdominal binding. This is an effort to bring the women's abdomen back to its normal shape without sagging as well as to avoid back pain.

"You bind the tummy with cloth to help make the body tight... When you are pregnant the tummy enlarges. You bind it so that the belly doesn't sag". (Tonusakhi, 38 years old)

5.5.1 Dietary Intake:

Till the fourth day they will eat rice cooked in an earthen pot locally termed as *kamuk* with salt and roasted fish. Pork/chicken soup is also given as it is believed that this will give a woman strength which is lost during the act of giving birth. Form the fourth day onwards they can start having plain, boiled vegetable. Rice will be cooked in the earthen pot. The spatula will be made of pine wood. Special care is taken that they are given boiled, warm water for drinking. While boiling water a piece of pine wood is added. They believe that pine tree has medicinal value for recuperation.

Women have assistance and support from husband, family members and neighbours. However there are also some women who don't have anyone. For these women, they try not to do "too hard" work but will attempt to carry on 'light' work around the house such as cooking and looking after the baby. However, this work should be undertaken at least ten days after the birth. Husband somehow take care and try to help out with the situation.

> "When you have a new baby, if you don't take rest then, later on it will cause you to have bad health". (Maibi).

This cannot be applied to everyone. So, women once they regain some strength do not lie idle on the bed. She starts lending a helping hand to household chores and other work even before three months of pollution is completed. However, she tries to avoid rigorous activity. It is believed that performing heavy activity can lead to *angang khao nanthaba* (prolapsed uterus).

> "If you lift heavy things then you will have *angankhaonanthaba.* It is like the womb collapse and comes out." (Shanti, 35 years old)

5.5.2 Avoidance of Sex:

Women also practice abstinence of sexual intercourse during this period. It is believed that intercourse during this period will cause *nupa mangba.* If a woman has this illness then her whole body will shrink and she will finally die.

5.6 CONTRACEPTION AND STERILIZATION

During the ethnographic phase, women did not mention about the indigenous method of controlling birth. One plausible reason might be the introduction of modern methods of contraception which is easily accessible. The National Family Program in its quest to introduce modern method of contraception all over India has wiped out indigenous methods of spacing and controlling birth.

The social and cultural practices which operate through the institution in this community assist in spacing birth and thereby limiting fertility to a certain extent. As Patel (1994) augments, "Rural societies do not just procreate on impulse and are in fact governed by definite indigenous modes of fertility control and not merely guided by an unrestrained biological instinct".

Abstention from sexual intercourse during menstruation and post partum period also plays a significant role in controlling fertility as it prevents couple form being together at the time of ovulation. In addition, sleeping arrangement also prevent couples from having the privacy to engage in sexual intercourse thereby contributing to prevention of conceptions. After having a few children, the woman often sleeps with the young children separates form her husband and thus prevent from conceiving.

Breast feeding practice too helps in widening birth intervals. Women continue breastfeeding the infant even after they start feeding them with other foods. This delays the onset of menstrual cycle and thus prevents a couple from conceiving.

Modern methods of contraception include female sterilization operation locally referred to as *hakchang semdokpa* (modification of the body) in Andro and operation in Kwakeithel. Few husbands of the women had undergone vasectomy. Some of the women had never used any contraception. A large number of women i.e. 45.9 percent of women did not use any contraception while in Kwakeithel only 28.4 percent did not use any contraception. The most commonly mentioned types of contraception in Andro are Copper-T, oral pill commonly known as Mala-D, and *hakchang semdokpa*. In Andro, 25.3percent of women reported using Copper-T. Two women complained of leakage of Copper-T .Some of the women have already taken out Copper-T as their husband complains of pain while having sex.

One informant in Andro cites:

"My husband took out the Copper-T. He scolded me for using it as it hurts him while having sexual intercourse." (Piktru, 35 years)

Another most frequently used contraceptive in Andro was oral pill with 16.0 percent of women, and 12.9 percent of women had undergone *hakchang semdokpa* (sterilization operation).

Table 5.1: Distribution of Contraceptive Users

Type of Contraceptive	Andro No. (%)	Kwakeithel No. (%)
None	89(45.9)	54(28.4)
Condom	0(0)	20(10.5)
IUD	49(25.3)	20(10.5)
Oral pills	31(16.0)	14(7.4)
Vasectomy	0(0)	3(1.6)
Tubectomy	25(12.9)	79(41.6)

Women in Andro did not report of using condom and vasectomy. In Kwakeithel the main methods of contraception is sterilization operation with 41.6 percent. However, fear always lurks around that an operation will weaken them and they will experience certain illnesses which they never experienced before. Intra uterine device and condom with 10.5 percent are the second most commonly used contraceptive. 7.4 percent of women in Kwakeithel use oral pills.

The above illustration on the usage of contraceptive and sterilization operation exhibits that women in Andro have more tendency to use intra uterine device and oral pills which they generally refer to as "mala-D". Sterilization operation is preferred less in Andro compared to Kwakeithel which might be because of inaccessibility of such facility in and around Andro. Compared to Kwakeithel, a large number of women did not report of using any contraceptive in Andro.

To surmise, this chapter describes the ways in which women in Andro and Kwakeithel perceive their bodies and body function. It presents women's belief and both observed and reported practices which affect their reproductive health status. These findings will create a backdrop for the locally perceived reproductive illnesses which will be presented in the consecutive chapter.

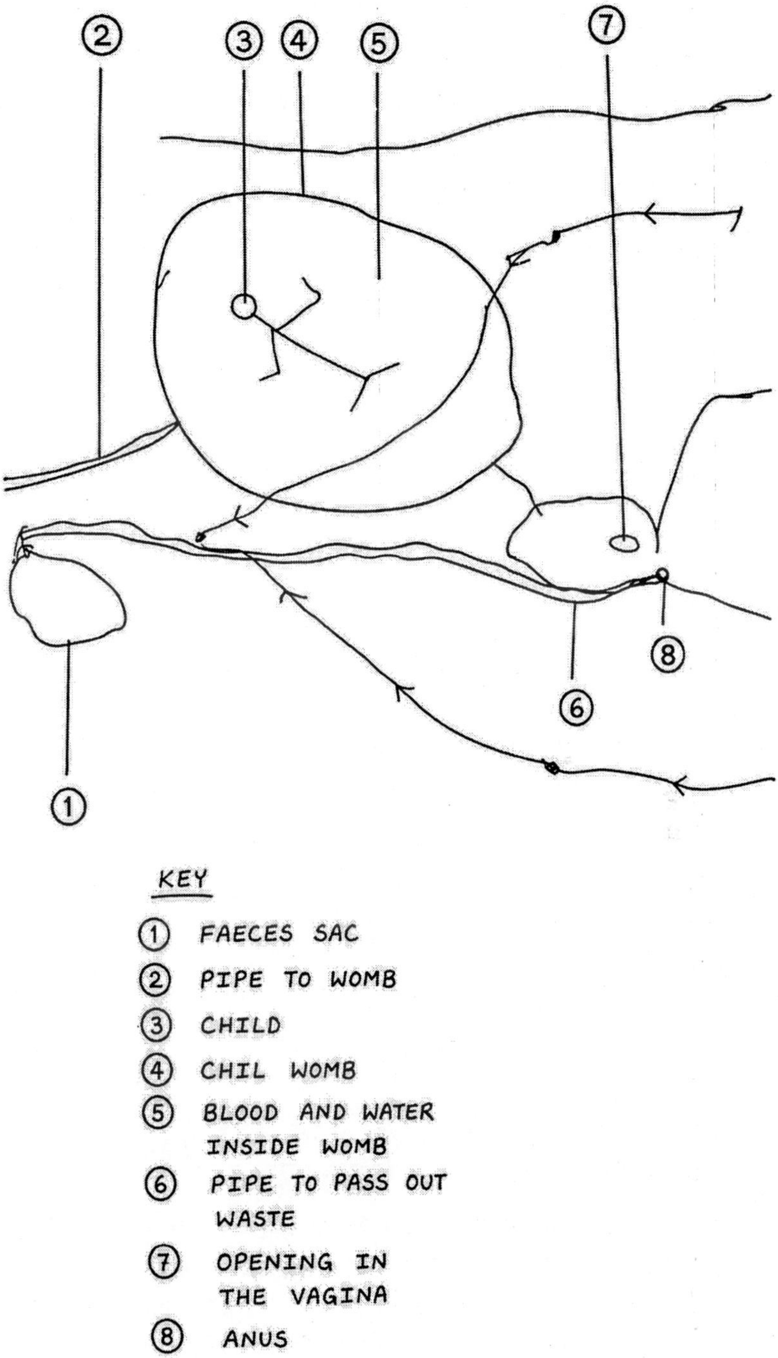

Figure 5.3: Close up of Women's Reproductive Parts on Body Map. (Traditional Birth Attendant

6

Women's Perception of Reproductive Illness and Their Health Seeking Behaviour

Perception of reproductive illness by the women themselves is important in understanding the women's reproductive health in a particular society. It also indicates the possibility of taking perception as a tool for measuring reproductive illness. This chapter presents rural Andro as well as peri-urban Kwakeithel women's perception of reproductive illnesses. In this section, all the illnesses/ problems which women perceive as *nupigi anaba* (women's illness), a plausible local denomination for "women's reproductive health problems/illnesses", have been presented. Women's perceptions of the seriousness of different women's illnesses are also described. The criteria for selecting specific women's illnesses for further investigation, symptoms and etiology of the three selected illnesses and a detailed ethno medical model of reproductive illnesses is presented in this chapter along with the treatment options for a particular illness.

Information presented in this chapter has been furnished from data collected in the ethnographic phase, as well as from data collected on symptom form of clinical samples. Ethnographic findings presented are those which women reported and which are observed.

6.1 NUPIGI ANABA (WOMEN'S ILLNESSES)

In Andro, while conducting interview with the *maibi's* (traditional birth attendant) and local healers in the community, certain illnesses were unraveled as experienced only by women. In Kwakeithel too, interviews with the women unveiled certain illnesses which only women experience. It explicitly shows that there are bouts of illnesses which only women experienced locally termed as *nupigi anaba* (women's illnesses) in both Andro and Kwakeithel and these symptoms of illnesses are not experienced by men.

During ethnographic study, women in both Andro and Kwakeithel spoke about several *nupigi anaba* (women's illnesses). Check listing of illnesses was compiled using the findings from free listing method as well as result from in-depth interview. This list was used to elicit information about each illness on symptom term descriptions, possible causes and health seeking behaviour.

The table below explicates the main *nupigi anaba* (women's illnesses) and was used to elicit information about each illness on symptom, term description, possible causes and health seeking Behaviour.

Table 6.1: Women's Illnesses

ILLNESS TERM	ENGLISH TRANSLATION	DESCRIPTION
Phingou Chatpa	White going	Vaginal discharge
Angangkhao nanthaba	Uterus coming out/body falling down	Vaginal itching
Mangbaga mari leinaba anaba - ee yamna chatpa mangba chang naidaba puk naba ee likna chatpa	Problems related with menstruation - blood oozing out irregular period stomach pain blood coming out stingily	Menstrual problem heavy period irregular period menstrual cramp scanty period
Khwang naba	Back pain	Pain at the back
Chaning naba	Abdominal pain	Pain in the pelvic region
Chakmangba / nupamangba	Rice polluted/man polluted	
Puk chakring	Stomach left over	Post delivery problem
kok ngaoba / Mit tandan paiba	Head spinning/seeing stars	Dizziness
Sonthaba	Weakness	Weakness

The free listing method showed that women perceived *Phingou chatpa* (white discharge) to be the commonest problem. *Sonthaba* (Weakness) and *mangbaga marileinaba* (menstrual problem) are also frequently mentioned illnesses indicating that these problems are among the most salient among women in Andro and Kwakeithel. However, the pile sorting method, focus group session and in depth interview with women revealed that *angangkhao nanthaba* (uterine prolapse) although, not reported with high frequency in the free listing results was a problem which women faced in silence until it disturbs their daily chores.

The local connotation for vaginal discharge is *phingou chatpa.Angangkhao nanthaba* refers to uterine prolapse and *Mangbaga mari leinaba anaba* refers to problems/illness related to menstruation. The reported menstrual related illnesses are- *ee yamna chatpa* (heavy menstrual flow), *mangba chang naidaba* (irregular menstruation), *puk naba* (menstrual cramp), *and ee likna chatpa* (scanty menstrual flow). *Khwang naba* (back pain) referring to pain on the back along the spinal cord. Most of the women face this problem of back pain several times in their lives.

6.1.1 *Chaning Naba* (Pain in the lower abdomen):

Chaning naba or pain in the lower abdomen is one of the problems which women in Andro and Kwakeithel face at different times of their lives. Some women say that they have this pain almost all the time. Some say that this pain is experienced when they work for long in the field or if they lift things which are heavy while others encounter it in their post-childbirth or post sterilization operation stage. Most women says that the pain surface up on cloudy days or on rainy days. Relief from this illness is achieved by massaging the abdominal and pelvic area with mustard oil and salt. In Andro, if the pain persists for long and becomes intolerable then they will call a *maibi/maiba* preferably a *maibi* for *puk suba* (massaging the abdomen). If this does not produce any effect then the woman will see a doctor in the nearest town.

In Kwakeithel, a woman will endure the pain by lying down or using hot water bottle or water bag and taking rest for some few days. If the pain becomes intolerable then they will gulp down one painkiller without doctor's prescription. However, if the pain persists then they will seek treatment from an allopathic provider. The most commonly taken drug when they have *chaning naba* was Ibrufen.

6.1.2 *Puk chakring* (Remnant blood):

Puk chakring is described as the pain which women experience after childbirth. Some of the key informants reported of women suffering from severe pain for several days after their last delivery. They were divided about the cause of such pain. Some said that the pain was basically due to *nungsit* (gas) because of the space created in the women's belly. They consider that pain wanes once the woman starts taking proper food.

Another interpretation is that *puk chakring* is due to incomplete cleansing of the blood which remains after giving birth to the baby.They believe that if the remnant blood remains inside the body for long then the concerned women will have unbearable pain in the abdomen. So if women have such kind of problem during post partum period then they seek treatment from the *maibi* (traditional birth attendant). The *maibi* will massage the abdomen chanting *mantras*. It is believed that the pain will wane after this enactment.

6.1.3 *Chak mangba / nupamangba* (Men polluted):

During post partum period if proper care is not taken then such illness often happen. Care should be taken properly regarding intake of her food and drinks during this stage and sex should be totally abstained. *Chak mangba* is the condition where the women will loose her tendency to eat. If these conditions prevail then she will puke even at the sight of food. People believe that it will get cured after some months. Care should be taken that during post partum a woman should drink only boiled water and use warm water. The water which becomes cold after boiling should also not be given because it is believed that this cause diarrhoea.

Nupamangba is the state which occurs when she had sex during post-partum period. In the first stage her face will get swollen up while her hands, feet and body will shrink. If she does not get any treatment then she will die after some months. People believe that even doctors cannot cure such ailments. It is only the *maiba's / maibi's* who can cure these types of illnesses.

Sonthaba (exhaustion) is an illness as well as the cause of other illnesses like *phingou chatpa* (vaginal discharge). Women often reported of *Chokthaba* or exhaustion in association with other illness as well as the cause of other illness. Women believe that the primary cause for these conditions is overloaded work and lack of nutritious food. *Kok ngaoba* (dizziness) is also another problem reported by women in both Andro and Kwakeithel but often in association with other illnesses. *Khwang naba* (back pain) is one major problem which most of the women in Andro are facing. Few women in Kwakeithel also reported of *Khwang naba* (back pain). Some have severe condition of *khwang naba* (back pain) that they have problem in standing up and sitting down. This illness is also associated with other illnesses. Women in Andro perceive that *khwang naba* (back pain) is due to heavy burden of circadian activities while in Kwakeithel women often associated *khwang naba* (back pain) with illnesses like *angangkhao nanthaba* (uterine prolapse).

6.2 WOMEN'S PERCEPTION OF THE SERIOUSNESS OF DIFFERENT HEALTH PROBLEM:

This section will discuss women's perception regarding the seriousness of three main illness which women in both Andro and Kwakeithel reported in higher frequency namely- *Phingou chatpa* (vaginal discharge), *mangbaga mari leinaba anaba* (menstrual problem), *angangkhao nanthaba* (Uterine prolapse). Women in both Andro and Kwakeithel believe that *sonthaba* (weakness) is the root cause of all the illnesses.

6.2.1 *Phingou Chatpa* (vaginal discharge):

Women's believe that an illness is serious for particular reasons. *Phingou chatpa* (vaginal discharge) is perceived as a problem when the discharge is an excess. In an in- depth interview -

> Thaba (a woman from Andro) said "If the discharge wets the *phanek* (wrap around) then the condition is serious"
>
> Shanti (a woman from Andro) said "When discharge falls a little it is okay but when it gets to be a lot then it is problematic"
>
> During of focus group session, Moyonsakhi (a woman from Kwakeithel) added: "If there is blood in discharge then it is a problem that needs to be looked into because it might be cancer."

Women use onomatopoeic terms like o-ro-ro chatpa (going), jo-ro-ro chatpa (going) to explain the severity of vaginal discharge. Women compare the severity of vaginal discharge allegorically with the menstrual blood flow.

"When the discharge is like the menstrual flow then it is a serious case". (Tampha, 34 years old woman from Kwakeithel)

Monsori (a woman from Andro) felt that women consider discharge a problem because:

"Women become weak and pale if they have this illness. It is not good to see women with *phanek* which is wet at the back. People might get some wrong interpretation".

From the above finding both in Andro as well as in Kwakeithel, women perceive that *phingou chatpa* (vaginal discharge) is serious when the discharge is in excess which they describe in onomatopoeic terms like o-ro-ro *chatpa* (going) or jo-ro-ro *chatpa* (going). The seriousness of *phingou chatpa* (vaginal discharge) was also described allegorically with the menstrual blood flow. They also perceive that *phingou chatpa* (vaginal discharge) is serious when there is blood in discharge.

6.2.2 *Mangbaga mari Leinaba Anaba* (Menstrual Problem):

Menstrual disorders are perceived as a problem with which women have to live and suffer. One of the menstrual problems which are perceived to be the most serious is heavy menstruation. They believe that heavy menstruation drains away all the strength and is considered to be weakening and cause dizziness and exhaustion.

In a focus group discussion session, Latitomala (a woman from Andro) responds: "Having heavy period is exhausting. This has been going on for last three months. When I have my period I cannot walk for long distance also. I feel weak and dizzy".

54 year old *maibi* from Andro commented: "Having heavy period after childbirth means that there must be some left over blood inside the body after giving birth. So, there is no harm in having heavy period. It is normal."

Though heavy period is considered a serious case, women in both Andro and Kwakeithel do not seek any treatment as they consider it normal. Menstrual disorders are perceived to be a problem which women have to suffer in silence. Moreover it does not disturb their daily ablutions so, menstrual disorder remains unattended.

6.2.3 *Angangkhao Nanthaba* (Uterine Prolapse):

Angangkhao nanthaba (uterine prolapse) were unanimously perceived by the people and *maibi's* which needs to be addressed by a doctor. Women in both Andro and Kwakeithel consider *angangkhao nanthaba* (uterine prolapse), a serious illness which needs medication from allopathic provider. They consider *angangkhao nanthaba* (uterine prolapse) serious when they see/feel the body parts coming out.

The *maibi* (traditional birth attendant) also put their hands up in such case. Monsori, a *maibi* in Andro commented:

"This is a serious problem because there is no treatment for this illness. One has to operate to lift up the *Angangkhao* (baby sac) at a big hospital which most of the women cannot afford. So, until and unless it disturbs the daily domestic chores one will not get treatment."

Women in Andro and Kwakeithel believe that many women suffered from *angangkhao nanthaba* (prolapse) but they suffer in silence because of the shame and stigma attached to this illness. Women in Andro believe that the only means is to push back the uterus inside. Moreover, economic crunch refrains women from seeking timely care.

Besides the three main illnesses - *phingou chatpa* (vaginal discharge), *mangbaga mari leinaba anaba* (menstrual problem), *angangkhao nanthaba* (prolapse) reported by women, other illnesses which are considered problematic are illnesses like back pain, abdominal pain, dizziness, weakness etc. Illness related with childbirth and pregnancies are not taken up for further investigation.

6.3 CRITERIA FOR SELECTION OF ILLNESSES FOR FURTHER INVESTIGATION

As this study aims to look at reproductive health problems a subset of women's non-pregnancy related reproductive illnesses was chosen for further investigation based on the following criteria of seriousness and commonness:

(1) Most frequently mentioned in the free listing results.

(2) Perceived that many women experience the illness.

(3) An illness which women are hesitant to report because of the

stigma associated with it and has been unattended to by health providers

Based on these criterions,–*phingou chatpa* (vaginal discharge), *mangbaga mari leinaba anaba* (menstrual problem), *angangkhao nanthaba* (prolapse) were looked into for further investigation for symptom, description, etiology and health seeking Behaviour for these illnesses.

Interviews with health care providers in Primary health center, Andro confirmed the selection of these women's illnesses for further investigation. They claim that women from Andro and from neighbouring areas come to Primary health center for seeking treatment for all same illnesses selected for this study.

Dr. Mani, MBBS who works at Andro Public Health Center describes the type of patients who come to him. "People come to me with seasonal illnesses like Diarrhoea, measles, cold. But women come all year round for vaginal itchiness, vaginal discharge, and menstrual problem and sometimes for pelvic inflammation. In Andro 40-50 have vaginal discharge and itching, 60-70 percent of women have menstrual problem. Dr Mani explained that he give treatment to women for discharge, itching and menstrual problem based on reported symptoms only. He further commented that the main cause of illness like discharge, itchiness is due to unhygienic condition of living.

Bhanu Puthem, working as a nurse in Primary health center, Andro for 10 years said that 80 percent who come for treatment in health center are women. There are many women in Andro who suffer from illness like vaginal discharge, itchiness, and who also have menstrual problem. 5 in every 10 must be suffering from such ailment. They do not come up until the problem disturbs their day to day activities. Women in Andro are too shy to open up and approach for the problem also.

Tamu Heikrujam who is working as a nurse in Andro Primary health center for 18 years believes that 50 percent of women have vaginal discharge. Uterine prolapse patients are less though may be 1 in 10 but the main problem is that women do not tell anybody about these problem. They do not say it directly. Only on being prodded do they state the gynecological problem. Andro women are too shy to come forward for such problem. Only when the condition becomes worse or unbearable they approach us.

6.4 THREE SELECTED REPRODUCTIVE HEALTH PROBLEMS

The three selected Reproductive health problems which are taken up for further investigation are: *Phingou chatpa* (Vaginal discharge), *mangbaga mari leinaba anaba* (Menstrual problems) and *angangkhao nanthaba* (prolapse)

6.4.1 *Phingou Chatpa* (Vaginal Discharge):

Phingou Chatpa literally translated as "white going" is frequently used to refer to vaginal discharge. Vaginal discharge is categorized into two types- non bloody and bloody discharge (*phingouda ee yaoba*). Women in Andro believe that when their body becomes weak they often have discharge. Bloody discharge describes the presence of blood in vaginal discharge. They believe that such a condition is serious and feel the need to attend to it properly.

Women have different perceptions about whom this illness affects and the extent to which *phingou chatpa* was prevalent in their village. In one focus group session women unanimously agreed that the illness was prevalent among sexually active women. Other women interviewed believed that *phingou chatpa* was prevalent among young unmarried girls, their neighbours and friend and estimated it to be between 40-50 percent prevalent in the village. In a focus group session Chingakham Tampaklei, 37 years old woman in Andro estimated the prevalence of *phingou chatpa* in the village to be 45-50 percent.

In a focus group session,

> Maimu Samjetsabam, a *maibi* rebukes "Even unmarried girls also have vaginal discharge. It is just that the family covers up because of the stigma associated with it. For every 100 women in our village 50 women must be having white discharge."

Though women reported of high prevalence of *phingou Chatpa* (vaginal discharge) they consider it as normal until and unless it disturbs their circadian activities. Women perceive that everybody have *phingou Chatpa* (vaginal discharge). The stigma attached to *phingou Chatpa* (vaginal discharge) also refrain women from talking openly about such illness.

Another responded:

"*Phingou chatpa* cannot be considered an illness until the discharge is too much that one cannot carry on with daily domestic chores. Everybody has it". (Thoibi 27 year's old woman from Andro)

An older key informant Leibaklei (a woman from Kwakeithel) said:

"It is not good for unmarried girl with wet *phanek* at the back. Their back is wet because they are *khatpa* (implying sexual intercourse)".

Young unmarried girl are chastised if people know that they have vaginal discharge. The basic indication was that vaginal discharge is associated with sexuality. Hence, only married women who are young and sexually active suffer from the illness. Some women furtively informed that unmarried girl also complain of this illness implying their involvement in pre-marital sexual interaction.

(i) Characteristic of *Phingou Chatpa* (Vaginal Discharge):

Women described vaginal discharge in terms of colour, smell, consistency, frequency and duration. Besides white discharge some women also complained of discharge with blood stain. They identified it as discharge with *laphutharo machu* (banana flower colour).

Discharge was easily distinguished in terms of texture: Women reported two types: 1) *eshinggumba* (Watery) 2) *nang nang laoba* (thick and curdy)

Smells are recognized by women particularly if the discharge were strong and foul which made women feel uncomfortable that other people may be able to detect it. Discharge with smell is described by women as *manam namthiba*(foul smell) women reported the presence of discharge without a smell as *manam namdaba* (odourless).

Women spoke of having large amounts or little discharge and were also able to describe the frequency which they had it i.e. they had it everyday or sometimes. Women also reported a range of duration for which they experience discharge problem. Some women said they have it before their menstruation for a few days. Illness narratives conducted on women who had reported *phingou chatpa* as an illness revealed the typical ways in which it is characterized.

"It is just like having menses. It soiled my phanek. I have to wear two phanek at a time" (Mema, 33 years old woman from Andro).

"It is white and has foul small. It itches a lot too. Whenever I go out I feel so conscious of the smell that I couldn't talk with my friends properly" (Thabalei, 32 years from Kwakeithel).

(ii) Etiology of *Phingou Chatpa* (Vaginal Discharge):

Analysis of ethnographic data revealed that women attributed *phingou chatpa* to several different causes. Causes listed in table below were most frequently mentioned by women in depth interview and in pile sorting of illnesses. *Sonthaba* (weakness), *wakhal waba* (worry), *asaoba* (anger), *thabak henba* (overload of work) conditions produced by economic hardship were felt to cause *phingou chatpa*. Eating fruits and avoidable food during menstruation and post partum period transform blood to water leading to *phingou chatpa*. Other factors believed to cause *phingou chatpa* were related to events like sterilization operation, wearing an intra uterine device, abortion and childbirth.

Table 6.2: Causes of *Phingou Chatpa* (Vaginal discharge)

Illness cause	English equivalent	Andro	Kwakeithel
Anangba	Poverty	√	√
Thabak kanna suba	heavy workload	√	√
Hakchang Phataba	Bad health	√	√
Cancer	Cancer		√
Sonthaba	Weakness	√	√
Maramchat oktaba nupi	An immoral women	√	√
Nupadagi Lounaba	Transmitted through male	√	√
Operation *toubadagi* / *Hakchang semdokpa*	After operation	√	√
Angang louthokpa	Abortion	√	√
Copper-T *happa*	Insertion of Cu-T	√	√
machi oiba chinjak watpa	Lack of nutritious food	√	√
Panty *setpa*	Wearing panty	√	√

During illness narrative interviews, women reported that the onset of *phingou chapta* occurred often because of one or more of these events. Some women who had *phingou chapta* at the time of interviewing said that they have no idea why they had this illness. Interview conducted with women provides examples of women's perception regarding the causes of such illness.

Sebomala Yumkhaibam, an older key informant from Andro explains:

"Now-a-days women do not put any restriction in their food intake during menses and post-partum period. They glutton up everything. It is because of this that blood turns to water and come out in the form of discharge."

Chingabham Tombinou, *maibi* in Andro retorts:

"Young women start wearing inners (Panties) which obstruct the circulation of the blood and causes many illness like vaginal discharge which is actually blood turned to water. Moreover, they do not restrict on tabooed foods which are supposed to be kept at bay during menses and post partum period".

Hemsori a *maibi*, 50 years old remarked: "*Phingou chapta* is the blood which actually turned to water because of carelessness in dietary intake during menstruation and post partum period."

"From morning till late night I don't have time to take rest for a minute. I have four sons and no daughter. There is nobody to lend me a hand. This makes my body so weak and *phingou* begins to fall". (Tonulembi 42 years old woman from Andro)

"Six year back I had *hakchag semdokpa* which makes me feel very weak and my body gets swollen up. After that operation *phingou* begins to fall". (Urirei 45 years old woman from Andro)

"Four months backs Copper-T was inserted in Primary Health Center. After that my husband keeps on complaining and since then I have had this problem". (Madhabi 35 years old woman from Andro)

"One year back I aborted one baby. Ever since then I have had this problem".

(Nganbi 37 years old woman from Kwakeithel)

Some women mentioned unhygienic way of living as a probable cause of vaginal discharge. Women in Andro associate *phingou chatpa* (vaginal discharge) with poor perineal hygiene and by working in dirty water in the rice field. To bring home the above said point the following verbose can be cited.

> Bhanu, a nurse in Andro says-"*Phingou Chatpa* in due to poor sanitation and unhygienic way of living."

> Memcha, 30 years old woman from Andro says," Discharge is caused by working in dirty water in rice field"

Women also relate their symptoms to different procedures or conditions that they had undergone. One woman in Kwakeithel attributed her vaginal discharge to pregnancy. Some blamed it on abortion and others claimed that *phingou chatpa* (vaginal discharge) is due to insertion of IUD. Women in Kwakeithel associate *phingou chatpa* (vaginal discharge) with cancer when a woman has discharge with blood stain.It happened when my third child was born. Right after delivery. (Bimola, 39 years old woman from Kwakeithel).

36 years old woman from Kwakeithel blamed her induced abortion for vaginal discharge:

> It is because of the induced abortion that I had vaginal discharge. (Noni 38 years old woman from Kwakeithel)

Another claimed Intra Uterine device (IUD) as the cause of vaginal discharge. Some women in Kwakeithel associate *phingou chatpa* (vaginal discharge) with cancer. When a woman has discharge with blood stain then she is suspected to be suffering from cancer. Some of the women perceive that *phingou chatpa* (vaginal discharge) can be transmitted from husband and can happen due to lack of nutritious food.

> "I think it is due to copper-T that I had put in. After putting that my vaginal discharge started". (Piktru, 42 years old from Andro)

> One woman in Kwakeithel responded:" I had discharge which is brick red/banana flower in colour for sometime and people say that it is cancer." (Gambhini, 37 years).

> Tampha 42 years old woman from Kwakeithel remarked: "Women also get vaginal discharge form men who got from other women"

> In the body mapping session, Leihao, 42 years old woman from

Kwakeithel described how this illness occurs: "*Phingou* comes from the place where menstruation blood comes from so, as long as one is healthy having all the nutritious food then the blood falls properly if not, then *phingou* will start falling."

"Women eat whatever is growing in their kitchen garden. They cannot afford to have nutritious food like milk, nuts etc to supplement their diet. Rice and curry are their staple food. This weakens a woman's body moreover a child bearing mother. Thus most women in Andro suffer from vaginal discharge."(Memcha, 37 years old from Andro)

6.4.2 *Mangbaga Mari Leinaba Anaba* (Menstrual Problem):

Mangbaga mari leinaba anaba (menstrual problem) a common complaint among women is a collective term for different illnesses / problems associated with menstrual periods. 27.3 percent of women suffer from menstrual disorder in Andro and 30 percent in Kwakeithel. Heavy menstruation was listed among 6.2 percent of the women in Andro and 6.3 percent in Kwakeithel. Women describe this as a debilitating illness which sucks out all their strength.

Chaobi, 30 years old from Kwakeithel describe:" I have been having menstruation with heavy flow. If I have menses then I feel very weak and dizzy that I cannot walk for long distance."

"If I have my menses then I have to lie down on my bed most of the time. I cannot do any work. Blood keeps falling and it never stops." (Sakhitombi, 28 years from Andro)

"Menstrual blood bleeds continuously and in abundance. All my *phanek* are soaked and it drips down my legs also. " (Satila, 33years old woman from Andro)

Menstrual cramp was reported in 2.6 percent of women in Andro and among 4.7 percent in Kwakeithel. Menstrual cramp was not considered as a serious illness. Women generally endure or bear the pain by lying down or using hot water bottle/water bag.

Ebechaobi Khumugmayum from Kwakeithel describes her menstrual pain: "I have menstrual pain on the first day of my period. On the 1st day I cannot do anything. I just lie down to bear the pain."

> Salam Lata, 34 years old from Andro says, "For five days I cannot do work properly. The pain stings me. When it shoots up my whole body shakes and I cannot get up".

Other menstrual problem like irregular menstruation and scanty period was also reported. Scanty period was reported only in Kwakeithel among 16.8 percent. Irregular menstruation was reported among 2.1 percent of women in Kwakeithel and 15.5 percent of women in Andro. In Kwakeithel, the frequency of scanty period reported by women is high. In Andro, women did not report scanty period. Women's report of irregular period was higher in Andro compared to Kwakeithel.

(i) Causes of *Mangbaga Mari Leinaba Anaba* (Menstrual Problems):

The causes of menstrual problem which women perceive include abortion, insertion of IUD, sterilization operation, pregnancy, delivery problems and improper cleaning during childbirth. Interviews with women provide examples of women's beliefs about the causes of menstrual problem.

> Hemsori 50 years old *maibi* from Andro reasons for menstrual problem: "If the remnant blood after delivering the baby is not cleaned properly then it happens"

> Another woman 45 years old woman from Andro describes the reasons for menstrual problem: "Women started putting foreign particle inside their body (copper-T) and had operation. All these block their tubes which lead to menstrual problem"

6.4.3 *Angang Khao Nanthaba* (Prolapse):

Angang khao nanthaba is literally translated as uterus coming out / body falling down. Women do not make any distinction between vaginal and uterine prolapses. They simply refer to a feeling of heaviness "down below" or that "something coming out" of vagina. Women believe that prolapse is an illness which needs attention from allopathic health care provider because there is no local treatment for it.

(i) Characteristics of *Angang Khao Nanthaba* (Prolapse):

Different types of prolapse that women experience are described. They have constant feeling of heaviness below or as if something is falling out from below making them difficult to sit, stand or walk. This makes them so inconvenient and disturbs their daily activities. This is associated with severe back pain. They cannot stand up abruptly after sitting also.

> Dhanapati Hijam (a woman from Andro) says "I had this illness two years back. I couldn't do anything during those days. My back was paining terribly and I can feel something heavy on my lower abdomen."

Prolapse interferes with women's work activities and with their lives. The degree to which they feel inconvenient by a prolapse depends on "how much the body is coming out". Women say that they have difficulty lifting weight, having sexual intercourse and difficulty in urinating when they have prolapse.

(ii) Cause of *Angang Khao Nanthaba* (Prolpase):

Women in Andro gave different version for causes of *angang khao nanthaba* (prolpase). Women believe that prolapse occurs due to long and difficult labour problem, carrying heavy items during post partum period, sterilization, frequent abortion and frequent childbirth. Interviews with women provide example of beliefs about causes of prolapse.

> "Frequent childbirth and abortion spoils the body. Playing with your body is not good. The pulling and pushing, inserting instruments and hand inside the delicate women's body will destroy everything." (Monsori, 43 years old woman from Andro)

During childbirth- if the foetus did not come out as soon as the amniotic sac burst then the maibi has to pummel the stomach and insert the finger inside the vagina to pull the foetus out. Simultaneously, the women is labour was encouraged to push harder to accelerate the birth of the child. Some woman remarked how this kind of pulling and pushing leads to prolapse.

Women also believe that lifting heavy weights also cause prolapse. In their day to day activities, a woman routinely lifts heavy weights. This includes lifting and carrying heavy pots of water from the ponds, hand pumps and tap to the house. Lifting heavy weight especially just after childbirth is considered to be dangerous because women's body during this stage is still tender and lifting heavy weight could push the body out.

It is believed that performing heavy activities can lead to a prolapsed uterus known as *angang khao nanthaba* as one woman in Kwakeithel relates: "If you lift heavy things during the post partum period when the body is tender after giving birth then you will have *angang khao nanthaba.* (Uterus coming out / body falling down). It is like the womb collapses and comes out. It is not painful but it is very uncomfortable."

Another woman from Kwakeithel incorporated: "I do not have anyone to look after the household so; before three month was completed after delivery I started working. I carried a potful of water and do all the household chores. Now, the doctors diagnose that I have uterine prolapse which is not severe."

Women also think that sterilization operation and inserting Copper-T (IUD) cause this problem because it weakens the body and makes it easier for the body to come out. Thus, women believe that problem during childbirth, lifting heavy weight or undergoing a sterilization operation are susceptible to *angang khao nanthaba* (prolpase).

6.5 AN ETHNO-MEDICAL MODEL OF NUPIGI ANABA (WOMEN'S ILLNESSES)

From all the data collected during ethnographic phase and survey phase what come up is the components of ethno medical model of women's illness. This model includes the root cause of women's illnesses and the intermediate causes.

6.5.1 Economic Hardship:

The cliché "No work, no pay" works in Andro and Kwakeithel. Women have to work hard to make both ends meet. There is also another saying in Andro and Kwakeithel -"If you don't work then you starve". Economic crunch in a household affect women. Engaged in a daily struggle to meet basic needs, they cannot spare time to improve and safeguard their own health.

Economic hardship compels a woman to work hard to meet both ends meet. This leads to physiological weakness, which in turn deteriorates the health condition and cause all the illness. The price of poverty has to be paid by women as poverty makes them compromise on their health.

> "I know that I could recuperate my illness if I have food but thinking about what my children will have if I spend on these foods I brush off even the idea of having good food." (Muni, 38 years old woman in Andro)

> "When a woman is pregnant or during post partum period a woman is supposed to be fed with nutritious and strengthening food but when you don't have the money to buy then you have to survive on whatever is available. This deteriorates the health condition of woman and invites all ailments." (Daya, 34 yrs old woman in Kwakeithel)

6.5.2 Susceptibility Determinants of Illness:

Women believe that when they are physically weak they are susceptible to other factors causing *phingou chatpa, mangbaga mari leinaba anaba and angang khao nanthaba.* These factors are referred to as "susceptibility" factors (Zurayk et al., 1993). These proximate factors may be categorized in the following manner for a general model of women's illnesses.

(1) Problem after sterilization operation or after insertion of Copper-T (2) Problem after a spontaneous or induced abortion (3) childbirth and delivery problem (4) Lack of nutritious and strength giving food. (5) Problem of violation of food taboo during menstruation and post partum period (6) Problem with transmission of illness through sexual intercourse from man to women (7) Lifting heavy weights.

There is a relationship between illness and weakness. An illness can happen to a woman via weakness. In the same parlance an illness becomes an agent of weakness.

> "When a woman is weak she is vulnerable to all illness." (Monsori, 24 years old woman from Kwakeithel)

> After inserting Copper–T, 5-6 months back I started having discharge "which makes me so weak that I feel exhausted now and then."(Thaba, 37 years old woman from Andro)

Thus illness and weakness have an undeniable interrelationship according to the perception of women in both Andro and Kwakeithel. They believe that when they are physically weak they are susceptible to factors such as insertion of Copper-T, abortion, childbirth etc. to cause illnesses like *phingou chatpa, mangbaga mari leinaba anaba and angang khao nanthaba.*

6.6 HEALTH CARE SEEKING BEHAVIOUR

Women reported an array of treatment choices for the three different illnesses, which ranged from no treatment to home remedies to visits to the doctor or hospital. Information were obtained from ethnographic interviews and from the symptom from filled in prior to a gynecological examination.

Majority of women in both Andro and Kwakeithel did not seek any treatment for all the three illnesses. In Andro 98.1 percent of women having menstrual problem, 53.7 percent of women with vaginal discharge and 91.7 percent of women suffering from prolapse did not take any treatment.

Among the women having menstrual problem only 1.9 percent had undergone home remedial treatment in Andro while in Kwakeithel 18.7 percent had undergone treatment especially self treatment.

For women who had *phingou Chatpa* among those who had undergone treatment majority i.e. 45.4 percent sought home remedies as treatment followed by 34.0 percent of women who sought treatment from maibi Andro. Few women (18.9 percent) sought treatment from an allopathic provider.

Looking at Kwakeithel majority (81.1 percent) of women sought allopathic treatment among those who sought treatment. Home remedies followed with (18.9 percent). For women who had *angang khao nanthaba* (prolapse).

The above results shows that majority of women did not seek treatment for vaginal discharge, menstrual problem and prolapse. Narrative interviews and focus groups session demonstrate women's perception on why they did not seek any treatment for these illnesses. Women often neglect their health until and unless the illness does not disturb them in their daily activities.

Because of the stigma and shame associated with vaginal discharge many women "hide" their problem. Women bear the brunt in silence and obscure the pain and suffering because of fear of social repercussion and stigma attached to such kind of illness.

> "For some, when they have vaginal discharge they are ashamed to approach health care provider for treatment so, they will wait until it becomes severe"

(Lalita, 38 years old woman from Andro)

Economic hardship was also features high on the list of causes which restrain women from seeking care. Financial constraints often become a hindrance in seeking timely care. Poverty compels both women in Andro and Kwakeithel to compromise on their health. They cannot avail themselves of the preventive health care or save themselves from the exigencies of the illnesses.

"I know that if I have milk and other nutritious food my problem *phingou chatpa* will be cured but who will feed me such things for free" (Sebomala, 27 years old woman from Andro)

Another woman who is 43 years old woman from Andro laments –

"I know that I have *angang khao nanthaba.* I am having problem in sitting and standing up but what will I do? If I go to a doctor, they will tell me to undergo operation for which I don't have money."

The prevailing fatalism about health problem, the beliefs that these conditions cannot be treated is also associated with women's limited awareness of their bodies and their reproductive system. Ignorance often endangers women's life. The belief that an illness is normal until it become severe often leads to hazardous end. Women often neglect and compromise their health until and unless the illness does not disturb them in their daily activities. The hazardous endeavour made by women to make both ends meet jeopardizes their health in many ways. The lifelong drain on physical stamina complicates the health of women.

Monsori, a traditional birth attendant emphatically said. "There is no treatment for *angang khao nanthaba.* I don't lay my hand on such case. I give treatment for vaginal discharge and menstrual problem only".

"I don't have time to go to the *maibi* or health center to seek treatment for vaginal discharge. Nothing happens to my body. Moreover everybody has it."(Thoinu, 37 years old woman from Andro)

Another recurring problem was the distance from health centre service and the problems of lack of transport to access the services in Andro. The sex of the health care provider too has a role to play in health seeking behaviour of women. In Andro, the doctor at the Primary Health Center is a male and for this reason women are reluctant to approach for such an illness.

"I don't want to show my private parts to a male doctor so; I do not go for treatment" (Leibaklei, 35 years old woman from Andro)

Some of the women who sought treatment follow a sequence of options ranging from self treatment or home remedies to visiting *maibi* (traditional birth attendant) on unqualified/qualified allopathic providers. Their choice of a particular treatment was based on recommendations from friends, relatives, or social contacts that had been successfully treated for vaginal discharge, menstrual problem or prolapse. However, women themselves were the final arbiters in deciding where to seek treatment.

6.6.1 Self Treatment or Home Remedies:

When women initiate treatment of all the three illnesses they always engage in self treatment or home remedies. Women were told of many home remedies either by their relatives or friends. Some of them were –

"I was told to sit on the hot water after boiling with *kangphan ekaithabi mana* for my *phingou*" (32 yrs old woman from Kwakeithel).

"Somebody told me to drink *ketuki mana* and *sitamishri* after boiling with water for vaginal discharge. After drinking this mixture my discharge stopped." (Saphabi 26 years old woman from Kwakeithel)

Other home remedies prescribed by women in Kwakeithel and Andro for vaginal discharge are drinking water of *komprek mana toutha* boiled with sitamishi, cooking *Lai Peruk* with *morok* and have it. In Andro, drinking water after boiling with *leiri* and *sitamishri* are believed to be good remedy for vaginal discharge.

In the verbose of one woman in Andro: "I have vaginal discharge associated with itching. It was so unbearable that I scratch it and have burning sensation. Even then also I was not satisfied so, I applied *yu machin* (local brew). Then, I got relief for some few days." (35 yrs old)

Thus, both in Andro and Kwakeithel, self treatment or home remedies are commonly sought for treatment of vaginal discharge. Depending on the availability of the resource the preference are given. Women in Andro mostly use *yu machin* (local brew) for vaginal discharge associated with itching as it is available in every household. However, *yu machin* (local brew) is not used in Kwakeithel as home remedial treatment.

6.6.2 *Maibi* (Traditional Birth Attendants):

In Andro, *maibi's* are sought for treatment of vaginal discharge and menstruation. They are mainly consulted for menstrual problem, though there are some cases of vaginal discharge. In Kwakeithel, *maibi's* do not have a role in the treatment of any of the three illnesses i.e. *phingou chatpa* (vaginal discharge), *mangbaga mari leinaba anaba* (menstrual problem)and *angang khao nanthaba* (prolapse).

> "I went to this *maibi* for irregular menses. She told me to sacrifice a black cock. I didn't do it as my mother-in-law forbade me to do so." (32 yrs. Old woman from Andro)
>
> Hemsori a *maibi* from Andro comments "Women come with all kinds of problems. I gave medicine prepared from herbs for vaginal discharge. They got better after drinking it."
>
> A 34 yrs old woman from Andro said, "I went to a *maibi* about one month back for vaginal discharge. She said she would give me some medicine. However, I couldn't go to collect it as my husband chided me. He told me to go to an allopathic practitioner."
>
> "I had watery discharge. I went to *maibi* for treatment. She gave me some potion to drink. After having it, I was fine and it never started again" (42 years old woman from Andro).
>
> "Whenever I have menstrual cramp the maibi does *puk suba* (stomach massage) and I get relief."(27 years old woman from Andro)

6.6.3 Unqualified and Qualified Allopathic Provider:

Women seek for medical intervention only when they find that they are too weak to work or when the condition is severe. Unqualified allopathic provider mainly points towards chemist. Majority of women in Kwakeithel seek treatment from allopathic provider while in Andro the trend of seeking treatment for these illnesses to an allopathic provider is new. For prolapse, they seek treatment only from an allopathic provider. Some women take medicine from chemist without any doctor's prescription.

> "I ask the chemist to give me medicine for vaginal itching and after using it I was fine."(32 years old woman from Kwakeithel)
>
> The different treatments that were prescribed to women by allopathic

practitioner were tablets, syrups, vaginal creams and passaries. Most of women did not know the name of the tablets and pills.

"I had bloody discharge. I went to doctor for treatment. He gave me medicine and it was fine for sometime but it started again. Now, I will go to hospital in Imphal." (A 35 yrs old woman in Andro)

"When I had discharge with itching the doctor gave me one cream to apply. After applying that it never came back" (32 yrs old woman Kwakeithel)

Doctor shopping is also found among women in Kwakeithel. In Kwakeithel, there is a plethora of private as well as government hospitals and clinics at furlong. So, women in Kwakeithel take advantage of the available facilities. Women look out for the most easily available, effective and cheap source of treatment and flock to that particular allopathic provider. Most of the women go for private allopathic provider or private clinics as they feel that it is easily available and the treatment is effective.

"I went to one doctor for prolapse. She gave me medicines but there were no symptoms of getting better so, I change the doctor. After getting treatment from her (the second doctor) I was cured." (45 years old woman from Kwakeithel).

"I went to the Doctor. He gave me some medicine. After that it got cured. I still feel the heaviness but it doesn't come out now". (Memcha, 38 years old woman from Kwakeithel)

Women in Andro visit the Primary health centre for vaginal discharge and menstruation but not for prolapse. Women believe that the only treatment for prolapse is surgery which can be done only at a hospital in Imphal. Therefore, they do not go to the *maibi* (traditional birth attendant) or the primary health centre for treatment of genital prolapse. Few woman in Andro reportedly visited hospital for all the three illnesses. Since going to the hospital involves expenses beyond their capacity women sought treatment only when one's condition becomes so severe that she cannot move and only if they can afford. The hospital is considered the only place they can approach for prolapse.

To surmise, most women sought no treatment for all the three illnesses– *phingou chatpa* (vaginal discharge), *mangbaga mari leinaba anaba* (menstrual problem)and *angang khao nanthaba* (prolapse).*Maibi* is one figure whom people feel comfortable and affordable for discharge and menstrual problem in Andro. Formal health care is sought only when the illness is severe and prevents a woman from performing her daily chores, in both the areas i.e. Andro and Kwakeithel. In Kwakeithel, seeking treatment from the *Maibi* (traditional birth attendant) is no longer in vogue. People go to government hospitals or private clinics for their treatment. In Andro, prolapse is one ailment which they believe could be treated only by undergoing surgery in hospital in Imphal. The doctor at the Primary Health Centre and *maibi* doesn't have a role in the treatment of such kind of illness.

To explicate or to drive home the women's perception of illnesses and their health seeking behaviour of women in Andro and Kwakeithel, the following cases has been taken up.

Case 1:

Kundalei is a 37 years old illiterate, very hard working woman residing in Andro who has a philandering husband. Her husband has a relationship with a widow- a mother of two children. She laments out how she quarrels with her husband about his philandering nature. She cannot leave him because of the growing up children. She gave birth to four sons and the youngest son is now nine years old. Her circadian activities starts early in the morning around 4:30 AM., and ends at late night around 10:00 PM. After getting up early in the morning she has to clean the surroundings of the house, fetch water, cook, and prepare her sons for the school. She looks after the rice mill as well as manages the household chores. Despite the hectic schedule she goes to the paddy field during sowing, transplanting, weeding, cutting, harvesting, threshing season.

After giving birth to the fourth son she aborted two babies- one in Hospital and one by the *maibi*. She underwent sterilization operation two years back. She was complaining of pain in the lower abdomen. She has *phingou chatpa* (discharge) associated with itching. She thinks that the discharge is because of the weakness after hectic schedule of the day's work.

She said that she don't have time to go to the *maibi* or doctor for the treatment. She tried some home remedies like sitting on the water boiled with *kangphan ekaithabi* but it did not help her. She blames everything on her misfortune and surrenders to God.

Case 2:

42 years old Pramo resides in Kwakeithel. She gave birth to four children and had undergone sterilization operation six years back. The eldest daughter is married. She is a housewife and her husband works as a government employee. Her husband is a diabetic.

She complains of frequent itching and *phingou chatpa* (discharge) at the time of the interview. Pramo said that the discharge started three or four months back. She believes that her husband did not have any sexual partner other than her. She takes bath regularly as well as abstains from sex during menstruation. Her menstrual hygiene also sounds to be good as she use only washed clothes and changed three or four times in a day.

Pramo did not go for any treatment as she thinks that the discharge is due to her bad health condition. She feels weak and exhausted most of the time. If she walks for sometime then she feels dizzy.

During the clinical examination she was found positive for Candidiasis which is commonly found among diabetes patient. She must have transmitted it from her husband so both Pramo and her husband were requested to take proper treatment.

Case 3:

Kaboklei is 45 years old woman who is tall, lanky and has five children. She hails from Andro. Before trying out the Copper-T and sterilization operation she had two abortions- both by the *maibis.* After that, she tried copper-T but her husband scolded her and she took it out. She had undergone sterilization operation four years back.

She was complaining of heaviness of the abdominal area and the sense of something coming out of her vagina while taking the case study. She also complains of severe back pain.

She said that her condition is the after effect of the heavy burden of work that she has to carry out during pregnancy and after giving birth and also due to poverty. She thinks that even if carry on the household work during post partum period if she had enough food then such a condition would not have happen. Kaboklei was also complaining of *miron leitaba* (no helping hand) so she has to do everything by herself. She said that she started doing household work with the baby slung on her back without even completing two months after giving birth. She also started brewing *yu* (local brew) to sell so that her children will not starve.She was also complaining about her husband who according to her is "good for nothing." He whiles away his time doing nothing.

She went to Andro Primary Health Center for treatment and the doctor diagnosed as *angang khao nanthaba* (prolapse) from the symptom that she described. The doctor gave her medicine but told her to go to RIMS (a hospital in Imphal). However, Kaboklei said that she don't have enough money to go to Imphal and undergo further treatment. She surrenders everything in the hand of God.

During the clinical examination she was diagnosed as having *angang khao nanthaba* (uterine prolapse) and referred her to RIMS for her treatment but she never visited the hospital.

Case 4:

Peiyobati is a tall, fair, fat woman of 40 years old staying in Kwakeithel. She divorced her first husband after giving birth to her son due to intolerable behaviour by the in-laws. She bought a land of her own and stays there. She got married with another married man and gave birth to a daughter.

Peiyobati was complaining of *phingou chatpa* (discharge) which she says is because of her bad health. Her second husband often pays a visit though he does not stay overnight. Both Peiyobati and her second husband are employed.

She said that her *phingou chatpa* (discharge) is watery but without any smell. She also said that the discharge is like the menstrual flow. She went to one private clinic but she was not satisfied with the treatment so, she was planning to change the treatment to another doctor for the treatment.

She indulges in sex during menstruation. She uses old rejected clothes as menstrual pad. She reuses the clothes after washing the cloth. The cloth is stitched on the panties and while washing and drying she does not take out the stitch.

She was found positive for trichomonas vaginitis. Both Peiyobati and her husband were given treatment and the first wife of her husband was asked to undergo treatment for the same.

Case 5:

Tampha, 45 years old is a school teacher residing in Kwakeithel. She has four children. After having four children, she aborted three times in a private clinic in Imphal. She tried copper-T but since it was not lifelong as well as it was painful so she took it out and underwent sterilization operation.

She had severe back pain, and heaviness of the abdominal area. She cannot sit and stand abruptly. She needs support to stand up. She went to one gynecologist for the diagnosis and treatment. The gynecologist diagnosed her as having prolapse and gave her some medicine which she was having.

Tampha believes that she is having *angang khao nanthaba* (prolapse) because of the rigorous activities that she has to do during post partum period. She cannot lie down and take rest for long because nobody is there to look after the household. Her husband helps her out in some ways but not all. She said that she used to carry water from the tap and started doing the entire household chores before completion of two months after giving birth.

Case 6:

Shanti is a 44 years old woman who never went to school. She was born and brought up in Andro. She was tall, lanky and has a charming face. She was cooking inside a smoke filled kitchen when the case study was in the process. Her house has three rooms, the middle one was kitchen cum sleeping room of the husband and wife. There was no chimney so; smoke was enveloping the whole room. Moreover, there was just one window. She was talkative so, both her hand and mouth were at work.

Shanti was complaining of *phingou chatpa* (discharge) with itching. She said that it is because of the sterilization operation. After that operation she has become thin and she feels that her body is shrinking. Sometimes, she scratches so she had burning sensation. Even then if she is not satisfied, she said that she pours *yu machin* (local brew) and tries to get some relief.

Regarding her menstrual hygiene, it was found that she used unwashed phanek and after wearing it she did not wash it properly. Due to water scarcity she tries to manage cleaning, washing with one bucket of water.

During menstruation she hardly takes bath and otherwise also she rarely takes bath. The place where she takes bath is on one stone slab just outside her hutment. She said that she cannot wash her vagina while taking bath because the bathing place is open and she cannot do so in the open.

Shanti thinks that her condition is normal because everybody has it. Moreover, she did not seek any treatment because she does not have money to buy medicine or get potion from *maibi* (traditional birth attendant)

Case 7:

Madhabi is a sweet young woman of 23 years old who got married just five months back after eloping with her long time boyfriend. She is happy trying to adjust herself with the new environment of unfamiliar faces. She was all decked up with bright colored clothes and jewellery.

She said that she has severe menstrual pain which happens almost every month, so fear always lurks around when her time for menstruation arrives. She said that the pain is almost unbearable. Moreover, she has heavy menstrual flow. She has the potion prepared by the *maibi* but sometimes it does not help her. If the pain is intolerable then the family members calls the *maibi.* The maibi conduct *puk suba* (massaging the stomach) which gives her relief. She did not go to an allopathic provider because she heard that taking allopathic medicine for menstrual problem will aggravates the problem.

During clinical examination, she was suspected of fibroid and referred to RIMS (Regional Institute of Medical Science) for further examination and treatment. She came once but the problem of distance, and after commuting for long having to wait for her turn to come compels her to stop visiting the hospital again. Moreover, it is a matter of money too so; she stopped going to hospital again.

This chapter has scripted out women's perception of their reproductive illnesses in Andro and Kwakeithel. Although women do not refer to such illness as "reproductive" illnesses, women are able to make a stark distinction of a group of illnesses which affect only women.

From the women's belief and reported behavior, an ethno-medical model of *phingou chapta, mangbaga mari leinaba anaba* and *angang khao nanthaba* is developed. This ethno medical model indicates that women perceive reproductive illnesses to be primarily due to lack of strength in their bodies which is brought about by economic hardships in a household. Women reported biological and behavioral causes, labeled in this ethno-medical model as proximate determinants of these illnesses, which affect them when they are weak. They believe that when their living condition is improved they will be able to improve their nutritional intake which in turn will strengthen them physically. If they remain weak then all sorts of illness will envelope them but if they are physically strong they can ward off illness.

Coming to health seeking behavior of women in both Andro and Kwakeithel, Andro has a kaleidoscope of health-care provider while Kwakeithel has variety of allopathic provider. In Andro, health-care provider includes- home remedies, *maibi* (traditional birth attendant) and the allopathic provider. In Kwakeithel, there is a plethora of allopathic provider which includes both private clinic as well as government hospital. Women in Andro find treatment given by *maibi* (traditional birth attendant) comfortable and affordable while women in Kwakeithel prefer private clinics which they consider as the most effective, easily available facility. Money and time involved in seeking allopathic provider compels women in Andro not to seek treatment, and satisfy themselves with the home remedial measures or the treatment given by *maibi* (traditional birth attendant).

A tapestry of case study has also been scripted in this chapter to illustrate the perception of the three frequently reported illnesses- *phingou chatpa* (vaginal discharge), *mangbaga mari leinaba anaba* (menstrual problem), and *angang khao nanthaba/hakchang mapan thokpa* (prolapse) and the health seeking behavior of women when faced with these illnesses.

7

Reproductive Morbidity: Women's Report, Clinical Examination and Laboratory Diagnosis and Associated Risk Factors

This chapter reflects on the results of the clinical phase of the study. The prime focus of this chapter is to compare women's reports with clinically and laboratory assessed condition. The correlation of clinical findings and laboratory diagnosis with a symptom can give the accuracy of the perception of symptom. It also indicates the possibility of taking perception as a tool for measuring reproductive morbidity. It is still an unanswered question whether women's self reports, the physician's clinical diagnosis or the laboratory examination independently can provide approximate estimation of reproductive illness. Therefore, assessment of reproductive illnesses was done using all the three technique. Determining the degree of association between women's report with clinical and laboratory diagnosis will be useful in determining the appropriateness of symptomatic treatment of gynecological conditions which is followed mostly by the Indian health providers in rural area. Women's perceived symptoms and clinical signs of reproductive illness are important tools of estimation of reproductive illness and their correlation with laboratory diagnosis helps in understanding the sensitivity of the signs and symptoms.

In Andro, women reported vaginal discharge associated with itching, weakness, backache, menstrual problem most frequently followed by general problems like digestive, circulatory/respiratory, nervous and sense organs in a range of 5-12 percent. Kwakeithel women follow the same pattern however there is comparatively lower prevalence of vaginal discharge associated with itching. In Andro, it is 47.4 percent while in Kwakeithel, 11.1 percent of women reported having vaginal discharge associated with itching. Weakness associated with fatigue/exhaustion is commonly reported by women from both the areas. The cases of infertility reported by women in Kwakeithel (12.1 percent) are higher than those reported by women in Andro (5.7 percent). Complaints about nervous/ sense organs, injury and skin problems are relatively less in both the areas.

Table7.1: Women's Self Reported Symptom and Respective Frequency in Andro and Kwakeithel

Women's self reported Symptoms	*Andro (N=194)* No. (%)	*Kwakeithel (N=190)* No. (%)
Discharge	104(53.6)	79(41.6)
Connective tissue	68(35.1)	78 (41.1)
Menstrual Problem:	53 (27.3)	57(30.0)
Heavy period	12(6.2)	12(6.3)
Irregular period	30 (15.5)	4(2.1)
Menstrual cramp	5(2.6)	9(4.7)
Scanty period		32(16.8)
Prolapse	36 (18.6)	28(14.7)
Digestive	23(11.9)	51(26.8)
Nervous/sense organ	20(10.3)	8(4.2)
Circulatory/Respiratory	14 (7.2)	22(11.6)
Urination problem	12(6.2)	9(4.7)
Infertility	11 (5.7)	23(12.1)
Post sterilization	10 (5.2)	6(3.2)
Infective /parasitic	8 (4.1)	12(6.3)
Injury	6 (3.1)	7(3.7)
Pregnancy and related problem	4 (2.1)	2(1.1)
Weakness	3 (1.5)	5(2.6)
Problem during intercourse	2 (1.0)	6(3.2)

7.1 WOMEN'S SELF REPORTED SYMPTOMS

In Andro, all the women who came for gynecological examination reported at least one symptom prior to clinical examination. 19.1 percent of women reported one symptom, followed by 28.4 percent of women who reported two symptoms, 22.2 percent reported three symptoms, 16.5 percent reported four symptoms and 13.9 percent reported five or more symptoms.

For Kwakeithel, woman complaining of two symptoms was highest with 38.9 percent and women reporting of five or more with lowest at 5.8 percent. In between are the women having three symptoms at 20.5 percent followed by women reporting four symptoms with 17.9 percent and women who reported only one symptom at 16.8 percent.

Table 7.2:
Frequency and Number of Women who Reported 0-5 Symptoms

No of Symptom	*Andro (N=194)* *No. (%)*	*Kwakeithel (N=190)* *No. (%)*
0	0 (0.0)	0 (0.0)
1	37(19.1)	32(16.8)
2	55(28.4)	74(38.9)
3	43(22.2)	39(20.5)
4	32(16.5)	34(17.9)
5	27(13.9)	11(5.8)

The most frequently reported illnesses are *phingou chatpa* (vaginal discharge) associated with itching, genito-urinary problems weakness, menstrual problem and connective tissue problems in Andro while in Kwakeithel *phingou chatpa* (vaginal discharge) is highest reported symptom *sans* itching. In Andro, 53.6 percent of women complained of *phingou chatpa* (vaginal discharge). Out of which, 47.4 percent of women reported of itching while 41.6 percent from Kwakeithel reported vaginal discharge prior to the gynecological examination.

Another most commonly reported cases of illnesses is genito-urinary problem with 35.6 percent and 27.4 percent followed by the connective tissue problem like body ache, backache which cumulates to 35.1 percent and 41.1 percent in Andro and Kwakeithel respectively.

Menstrual problem is also commonly reported by women from both the areas. 27.3 percent of women complained of menstrual problem prior to clinical examination in Andro and 30.0 percent in Kwakeithel. Out of these women, the most frequently reported menstrual problem is irregular period with 15.5 percent in Andro, while in Kwakeithel; it is scanty period with 16.8 percent. Other menstrual problems reported are heavy period and pain during menstruation. The general associated problems with menstruation are weakness, body ache and dizziness.

7.1.1 Check Listing of the Self Reported Symptoms of Illnesses

Table 7.3: Frequency after Check Listing of Self Reported Symptoms

Illness	*Self reported*		*Additional when check listed*		*Total*	
	Andro (N=194) No.(%)	*Kwakei-thel (N=190) No.(%)*	*Andro (N=194) No.(%)*	*Kwakei-thel (N=190) No.(%)*	*Andro (N=194) No.(%)*	*Kwakei thel (N=190) No.(%)*
Phingou chatpa (vaginal discharge)	68(35.1)	57(29.3)	36(18.5)	22(11.3)	104(53.6)	79(41.6)
Mangbaga mari leinaba anaba. (menstrual problem)	41(21.1)	47(24.7)	12(6.2)	53 (10)	53(27.3)	57(30.0)
Phinungi oiba anaba (sexual problems)	2(1.1)	5(32.2)	98(50)	73(38.4)	99(51.1)	79(41.6)
Angangkhao nanthaba/ hakchang mapan thokpa nanthaba (prolapse)	13(6.7)	22(11.6)	23(11.9)	16(3.2)	36(18.6)	28(14.7)

Women's reproductive health encompasses certain dimensions which are sensitive and needs to be handled with tact. An account with the women during ethnographic phase unraveled that women were more open about certain reproductive illnesses/symptoms such as vaginal discharge or menstrual problem when compared to certain issues which pertains to problem during sexual intercourse. These issues need to be open up. When prompted a large number of women mentioned about symptoms they had not self-reported earlier. Thus, checks listing of reported symptoms of illness enable to elicit the obscured reproductive illnesses that women had. Most of the women were embarrassed to report their ailments.

When women were prompted there is an increase in the frequency of the reported problems about vaginal discharge, itching, menstrual problems, prolapse, problem during sexual intercourse and infertility problem. Very few people reported about problem during sexual intercourse. Women report about their problems when they are prompted. In Andro 50 percent of the women were found having sexual problem when prompted while in Kwakeithel, 38.4 percent were added when check listed. This might be because of the fact that women in Andro were more conservative in their outlook and were more conscious of being reprimanded because of the stigma attached to such type of problem. At the same parlance is the case of prolapse where 11.9 percent of women were found suffering from prolapse when check listed. In Kwakeithel, 3.2 percent of women were added after check listing which is comparatively lower. However, women are more willing to report reproductive illnesses like vaginal discharge associated with itching, menstrual problem. Thus, it is overt that women perceive such kind of reproductive illnesses as common among them and hence do not hesitate to report to a health provider. On the other hand, problems about sexual intercourse which is associated with their sexual anatomy and function, women are not comfortable in disclosing unless prompted.

7.2 CLINICAL EXAMINATION AND PREVALENCE OF RELATED MORBIDITIES

In this section, the diagnostic criteria and the prevalence of gynecological morbidities clinically examined by the gynaecologist and by simple laboratory test and pap smears are presented.

7.2.1 Criteria for Clinical Diagnosis:

The clinical entities were diagnosed as per standard criteria. This section describes the criteria used for clinical and laboratory diagnosis of morbidities as described by standard gynaecology textbooks (Tindall, 1993).

(1) Vaginitis: Complaint and presence of abnormal discharge during examination. The discharge was described in terms of amount, colour and consistency and its association with itching.

Microscopically discharge with ≥ 5 pus cells per high power field was also considered as abnormal.

(ii) Cervicitis: Presence of cervical erythema (inflammation) and mucopurulent discharge.

Microscopically presence of cervical pus cells ≥ 10 per high power field in women with cervical discharge.

(iii) Cervical Erosion: A bright red clearly defined area on the vaginal aspect of the cervix where squamous epithelium is replaced by columnar epithelium.

(iv) Pelvic Inflammatory Disease: Presence of abdominal tenderness and uterine tenderness with or without adnexal tenderness.

(v) Prolapse: Confirmed by direct examination

Rectocoele Prolapse: Descent of posterior vaginal wall below its normal position.

Cystocoele Prolapse: Descent of anterior vaginal wall below its normal position.

Uterine Prolapse: Descent of the uterus below its normal position.

(vi) Laboratory Diagnosis Criteria:

Candidiasis: Presence of hyphae and spores on direct microscopy of KOH mount preparation.

Bacterial Vaginosis: Positive whiff test a fishy odour when KOH is added to the discharge. Vaginal pH measurement ≥ 5 and direct microscopy of "clue cells".

Trichomoniasis: Presence of motile protozoa during direct microscopy of saline wet mount.

7.2.2 Reproductive Morbidity Assessed by Clinical Examination and Laboratory Methods:

Women's reproductive morbidity was assessed by using clinical and simple laboratory test. In Andro clinical examination as well as laboratory results shows that 23.2 percent of women had vaginitis. In Kwakeithel, on clinical examination, 17.4 percent of women were found having vaginitis. When examined using laboratory method, 17.9 percent of women were found to have vaginitis. Laboratory assessment of the individual vaginal infection shows 7.7 percent and 6.3 percent of women having candidiasis in Andro and Kwakeithel. 13.7 percent and 9.5 percent of women had bacterial vaginosis while 2.6 percent and 2.1 percent of women were found to have trichomoniasis in Andro and Kwakeithel.

In Andro, 10.3 percent i.e. 20 women were identified having PID while in Kwakeithel only 2.6 percent i.e. 5 women were diagnosed having PID. It is hypothesized that PID may be prevalent in women due to previous lower reproductive tract and/or as infections which may be introduced through procedures like childbirth, abortion and sterilization operation.

Table7.4: Prevalence of Gynecological Morbidities (Clinical and Laboratory Diagnosis)

Morbidity	*Andro (N=194)* No. (%)	*Kwakeithel (N=190)* No. (%)
Clinical Vaginitis	45(23.2)	33(17.4)
Vaginitis by laboratory tests	45(23.2)	34(17.9)
Candidiasis	15(7.7)	12(6.3)
Bacterial Vaginosis	26(13.7)	18(9.5)
Trichomoniasis	5(2.6)	4(2.1)
Clinical Cervicitis	26(13.4)	19(10.0)
Pelvic Inflammatory Disease	20(10.3)	5(2.6)
Cervix erosion	14(7.2)	9(4.7)
Prolapse	52(26.8)	23(12.1)
Rectocoele	3(1.5)	1(0.5)
Cystocoele	9(4.6)	1(0.5)
Cystocoele and Rectocoele	19(9.8)	12(6.3)
Cystocoele and uterine	8(4.1)	1(0.5)
Uterine and Vaginal	9(4.6)	5(2.6)
Uterine only	5(2.6)	3(1.6)

Cervical screening is an important parameter of reproductive health. Clinically, cervical erosion was detected in 6.7 percent (13) of women in Andro and among 4.7 percent (9) women in Kwakeithel. The gynaecologist diagnosed a woman with cervical ectopy only when she observed an ectopy on the cervix where the squamous epithelium is replaced by columnar epithelium and has a bright red, clearly defined area on the vaginal aspect of the cervix. Although cervical ectopy is not considered as abnormal many physicians still believe that an ectopy might result after an infection and continue to diagnose this condition (Tindall, 1993). 13.4 percent of women were found to be clinically positive for cervicitis in Andro while in Kwakeithel 10.0 percent of women were detected having cervicitis.

The prevalence of genital prolapse is more among women in Andro than the women in Kwakeithel, 26.8 percent and 12.1 percent of women in Andro and Kwakeithel showed at least one type of genital prolapse. 2.6 percent and 1.6 percent of women in Andro and Kwakeithel respectively had uterine prolapse only. 1.5 percent and 4.6 percent of women in Andro had only rectocoele and cystocoele. In Kwakeithel, the prevalence of only rectocoele and cystocoele was 0.5 percent. 4.1 percent in Andro and 0.5 percent of women in Kwakeithel were detected having cystocoele (anterior vaginal prolapse) and a uterine prolapse. In Andro, 4.6 percent of women and 2.6 percent of women in Kwakeithel had cystocoele, rectocoele and uterine prolapse.

During clinical examination, 25.8 percent of women were found to be free from gynecological morbidities in Andro. In Kwakeithel, the frequency of women with no gynecological morbidities was 53.2 percent which is comparatively high. 35.6 percent and 27.9 percent of women in Andro and Kwakeithel had one morbidity followed by women having two morbidities which are 26.8 percent and 15.8 percent respectively in Andro and Kwakeithel. 8.8 percent and 1.1 percent of women in Andro and Kwakeithel had three morbidities. 2.1 percent and 1.0 percent of women in Andro were diagnosed having four and five gynecological morbidities while 1.1 percent each was found having four and five gynecological morbidity in Kwakeithel.

Table7.5: Number of Morbidities and Frequency in Andro and Kwakeithel

Number of morbidities	*Andro* *no. (%)*	*Kwakeithel* *no. (%)*
0	50(25.8)	101(53.2)
1	69(35.6)	53(27.9)
2	52(26.8)	30(15.8)
3	17(8.8)	2(1.1)
4	4(2.1)	2(1.1)
5+	2(1.0)	2(1.1)

7.2.3 Perceived Morbidity, Clinical Findings and Laboratory Diagnosis:

The table given below summarizes the gynecological morbidities and the instruments that are used to measure the gynecological and related morbidity including women's self reported symptoms, a clinical examination and laboratory testing. However, these three instruments could not be applied to all the disease elements. On the one hand, only some of the selected disease elements have expected symptoms that can be recognized by women like discharge and prolapse which are obvious with specific physical symptoms. On the other hand, conditions take PID and cervical ectopy were not necessarily articulated by women using local term because they are asymptomatic and thus do not have any physical symptoms that are associated with them. These conditions fall within the paradigm of medical examination taken up by the gynaecologist/ physician. These conditions are more obvious to a physician who has the capacity to visualize clinical findings in the vagina and cervix at the time of examination.

Vaginitis was diagnosed using clinical and laboratory methods as well as by evaluating the symptoms reported by women. Cervicitis, Pelvic inflammatory disease and cervical ectopy were assessed only by clinical examination. Cervicitis may be confirmed with laboratory test which involve cervical swab culture, gram staining or fluorescence microscopy. However, due to resource constraints these tests could not be done for this study. Infertility, menstrual problem could only be assessed through women's reported symptoms. Prolapse was assessed using both women's reports of *Angang khao nanthaba/hakchang mapan thokpa* and clinical examination. If morbidity is assessed by more than one method, a comparison of the methods is presented below-

Table 7.6: Gynecological Morbidity and Method Used

Gynecological morbidity	*Women's self reports*	*Clinical examination*	*Laboratory Test*
Vaginitis	X	X	X
Cervicitis	*	X	
PID	*	X	
Cervical ectopy	*	X	
Prolapse	X	X	

Gynecological morbidity	*Women's self reports*	*Clinical examination*	*Laboratory Test*
Menstrual problem	X		
Problem with intercourse	X		
Infertility	X		

X denotes that this method was used in this study

* denotes lack of local terminology which describe this specific a condition

Throughout a women's reproductive span, vaginal discharge remains to be the commonest problem and an enroute towards reproductive tract infection. In this study, the most frequently reported symptom i.e. vaginal discharge will be used for the diagnosis of reproductive tract infection. Women's self reports were compared with gynecological observation of presence of vaginal discharge.

(i) *Comparison of Women's Report of Phingou Chatpa and Gynaecologist Observation of Presence of Vaginal Discharge*

Table 7.7: Women's Report and Gynecological Observation of Vaginal Discharge

Women's Report of Phingou Chatpa	*Andro*		*Total*	*Kwakeithel*		*Total*
	vaginal discharge			*vaginal discharge*		
	Present	*Absent*		*Present*	*absent*	
present	69	35	104	43	36	79
absent	13	77	90	2	109	111
Total	82	112	194	45	145	190

Area	*Sensitivity (%)*	*Specificity (%)*	*PPV (%)*	*NPV (%)*	*Agreement (%)*	*Kappa*
Andro	84.1	68.8	66.3	85.5	75.2	0.509
Kwakeithel	95.5	75.2	54.4	98.2	80	0.559

In Andro, the gynaecologist detected the presence of vaginal discharge in 82 women, 69 of these women reported *phingou chatpa* prior to the examination. The gynaecologist observed no discharge among 112 women. However 35 women reported the presence of *phingou chatpa.*

While the gynaecologist observed the presence of vaginal discharge among 45 women, 43 women reported of *phingou chatpa* prior to clinical examination in Kwakeithel 145 were observed negative presence of vaginal discharge by the gynaecologist of whom 36 women reported of *phingou chatpa.*

Sensitivity, specificity, positive predictive value, negative predictive value, percentage of agreement and Kappa were used for comparison.

The formula for kappa (K) used is

$$K = \frac{\text{\% observed agreement - \% agreement expected by chance}}{\text{100\% - \% agreement expected by chance}}$$

The predictive value of reported symptoms was considered important because it provides information about the relative magnitude of accurate positive and negative predictions from women's report and gynecological examination.

There was significant association between the presence of *phingou chatpa* reported by women vis-à-vis women diagnosed having vaginal discharge by the gynaecologist. Both sensitivity and specificity are fairly high with 84.1 percent and 68.8 percent in Andro and 95.5 percent and 75.2 percent in Kwakeithel. The negative predictive value was 85.5 percent and 98.2 percent in Andro and Kwakeithel.

The positive predictive value i.e. percentage of women who reported *phingou chatpa* and in whom the discharge was observed by the gynaecologist were 65.4 percent and 54.4 percent in Andro and Kwakeithel. The agreement was 75.2 with a kappa of 0.509 in Andro and an agreement percent of 80 with a kappa of 0.568 in Kwakeithel which indicates a moderate concordance between women's report of *phingou chatpa* and gynaecologist's observations for the presence of discharge in Andro and in Kwakeithel.

The moderate concordance in Andro and Kwakeithel might be because of the following stated reasons:

(i) women must have reported the presence of *phingou chatpa* from recent but not a current episode of morbidity

(ii) women might report of *phingou chatpa* as an illness which does not mean a physical symptom of discharge to them.

(i) women may have cleaned themselves prior to examination.

(ii) *Comparison of Women's Report of Phingou Chatpa and Gynaecologist's Diagnosis of Vaginitis/Cervicitis*

Table 7.8: Women's Report and Gynaecologist Diagnosis of Vaginitis/ Cervicitis

Women's Report of phingou chatpa	*Andro*			*Kwakeithel*		
	vaginitis/cervicitis			*vaginitis/cervicitis*		
	present	*absent*	*Total*	*present*	*absent*	*Total*
present	40	64	104	35	44	79
absent	8	82	90	0	111	111
Total	48	146	194	35	155	190

Area	*Sensiti-vity (%)*	*Specificity (%)*	*PPV (%)*	*NPV (%)*	*Agree-ment (%)*	*Kappa*
Andro	83.3	56.1	38.5	91.1	62.9	0.29
Kwakeithel	100	76.6	44.3	100	76.8	0.48

Similar trend follows when women's report of *phingou chatpa*is compared with gynaecologist's clinical diagnosis (observation of abnormal discharge and inflammation of the vagina and or cervix) of vaginitis and/ or cervicitis. The positive predictive value for Andro and Kwakeithel are 38 percent and 44.3 percent.

Sensitivity was high due to high report of *phingou chatpa* in Andro (83.3 percent) and Kwakeithel (100 percent. The comparison between women's report of *phingou chatpa* and the clinical diagnosis of an infection shows fair level of concordance (agreement =62.9 percent and kappa =0.29) between the two measures in Andro and moderate level of concordance (agreement =76.8 percent and kappa =0.48) in Kwakeithel. The moderate specificity results from the fact that women reported *phingou chatpa* when they did not have abnormal discharge due to an infection in the cervix and vagina. The low positive predictive value in both the areas might be because of the following stated reasons: women must have reported the presence of *phingou chatpa* from recent but not a current episode of morbidity, women might report of *phingou chatpa* as an illness which does not mean a physical symptom of discharge to them, women may have cleaned themselves prior to examination.

(iii) *Comparison of Women's Report of Phingou Chatpa and Laboratory Diagnosis of Vaginitis*

Table 7.9: Women's Report and Laboratory Diagnosis of Infection.

Women's self Report of phingou chatpa	*Laboratory Diagnosis*					
	Andro vaginitis			*Kwakeithel vaginitis*		
	present	*absent*	*Total*	*present*	*absent*	*Total*
present	36	65	101	34	44	78
absent	9	80	89	0	109	109
Total	45	145	190	34	153	187

Area	*Sensiti-vity (%)*	*Specificity (%)*	*PPV (%)*	*NPV (%)*	*Agree-ment (%)*	*Kappa*
Andro	80	55.2	35.6	89.9	61.1	0.247
Kwakeithel	100	71.2	43.6	100	76.5	0.474

Women's report of *phingou Chatpa* was also compared to the laboratory diagnosis of infection. This comparison unraveled a fairly high sensitivity (80 percent) and moderate specificity (55.2 percent) of *phingou chatpa* in Andro and an equally very high sensitivity (100 percent) and high specificity (71.2 percent) of *phingou chatpa* in Kwakeithel. The positive predictive value in Andro and Kwakeithel are 35.6 percent and 43.6 percent.

The women's reported symptoms of *phingou chatpa* with laboratory diagnosis in Andro has agreement of 61.1 percent with kappa of 0.247 and an agreement of 76.5 percent with kappa value of 0.474 in Kwakeithel. This indicates that in Andro, *phingou chatpa* is not a good predictor of the presence of vaginal discharge and a moderate predictor in Kwakeithel.

However, the low concordance in Andro and moderate concordance in Kwakeithel might be due to lack of more sophisticated laboratory methods which could detect the presence of pathogens responsible for infection like Chlamydia, Gonorrhea and not just limiting laboratory diagnosis to *Trichomonas vaginitis, Bacterial vaginitis* and *Candida* due to lack of resource.

(iv) *Comparison of Gynaecologist's Diagnosis of Vaginitis/Cervicitis and Laboratory Diagnosis of Vaginitis*

Table 7.10: Gynaecologist's Diagnosis of Vaginitis/Cervicitis and Laboratory

Gynaecologist's diagnosis of vaginitis/ cervicitis	*Laboratory Diagnosis*					
	Andro			*Kwakeithel*		
	vaginitis			*vaginitis*		
	present	*absent*	*Total*	*present*	*absent*	*Total*
Present	45	3	48	34	1	35
Absent	0	142	142	0	152	152
Total	45	145	190	34	153	187

Area	*Sensiti-vity (%)*	*Specificity (%)*	*PPV (%)*	*NPV (%)*	*Agree-ment (%)*	*Kappa*
Andro	100	97.9	93.8	100	98.4	0.056
Kwakeithel	100	99.3	97.1	98.1	99.4	0.98

Diagnosis of Vaginitis

To check the validity of the clinical diagnosis of lower Reproductive tract Infections (RTI) with the laboratory diagnosis the following analysis was carried out. Sensitivity was high as all 45 women and 34 women in Andro and Kwakeithel who were diagnosed by the gynaecologist as having vaginitis or cervicitis had infection on laboratory result. Specificity was also high with 97.9 percent and 99.3 percent in Andro and Kwakeithel. Positive predictive value and negative predictive value are also high in both the areas.

To surmise, women's report of *phingou Chatpa* has high sensitivity. However, it is not a good predictor of lower vaginal and cervical infections. Clinical diagnosis however agrees with simple laboratory diagnosis.

(v) *Comparison of Women's Report of Angang khao Nanthaba/Hakchang Mapan Thokpa and Gynaecologist's Observation of any Prolapse*

Table 7.11: Women's Report of *Angang khao Nanthaba/Hakchang Mapan Thokpa* and Gynaecologist's Observation of any Prolapse

Women's self report of Angangkhao nanthaba/ hakchang mapan thokpa	*Gynaecologist's observation*					
	Andro			*Kwakeithel*		
	prolapse			*prolapse*		
	present	*absent*	*Total*	*present*	*absent*	*Total*
Present	25	11	36	22	6	28
Absent	27	131	158	1	161	162
Total	52	142	194	23	167	190

Area	*Sensitivity (%)*	*Specificity (%)*	*PPV (%)*	*NPV (%)*	*Agreement (%)*	*Kappa*
Andro	48.1	92.3	69.4	82.9	94	0.83
Kwakeithel	95.6	96.4	78.5	99.3	96	0.82

This section discusses about the symptom/illness like *angang khao nanthata/hakchang mapan thokpa* (uterus falling out/body coming out) which is recognized by a woman if it is visible or feel it. Comparison of this local terminology with the clinical diagnosis of prolapse shows that sensitivity of this term is low in Andro (48.1 percent) while it is high in Kwakeithel (95.6 percent).

The low sensitivity in Andro might be explained by the cases of 27 women who did not report the symptom of prolapse but clinically diagnosed having prolapse. On further examination, out of these 27 women 21 were found having only vaginal prolapse, that are neither visible to women nor felt by women to be able to report it while the remaining were found having uterine prolapse. On further questioning, they said that they were embarrassed to talk about it.

Specificity of local term is high in both Andro (92.3 percent) and Kwakeithel (96.4 percent). Women's report of "uterus falling out/body coming out" shows a higher concordance with the clinical diagnosis of prolapse and appears to be a good predictor of prolapse in Andro with positive predictive value of 69.4 percent as well as in Kwakeithel (PPV = 78.5 percent). The degree of agreement is high in both Andro and

Kwakeithel with 94 percent and 96 percent respectively. The concordance between women's report of *angang khao nanthaba/hakchang mapan thokpa* (uterus falling out/body coming out) and gynecological observation is very good in Andro (Kappa =0.83) and Kwakeithel (Kappa =0.82). This culminates that *angang khao nanthaba/hakchang mapan thokpa* (uterus falling out/body coming out) is a good predictor of genital prolapse.

7.2.4 Predictors of Reproductive Tract Infection and Genital Prolapse:

This section deals with the correlation of numerous potential risk factors with reproductive tract infections and genital prolapse. The following potential risk factors were analyzed for correlation with the infections and genital prolapse: (1) socio-economic factors (2) Personal hygiene (3) Menstrual practices and hygiene (4) Obstetric factors (5) Family planning practices.

To determine the risk factors for reproductive tract infection the following variables are taken up:

Socio-economic factors have the following independent variables: age, age at marriage, type of family, relation of the women with the head of the household and total family income per month.

Personal hygiene include variables like taking bath daily, place of taking bath, washing private parts; changing undergarments if not taken bath, washing hand before eating, boiling of drinking water and washing hand after defecation.

Menstrual practices and hygiene has independent variables like type of material used, during menses, number of clothes changed in the first two days, washing private parts and awareness of reproductive tract infections.

Obstetric factor includes variables like number of children, place of birth of last baby, person conducting the delivery, material used for cutting chord, person and place where abortion/still birth was conducted. Type of contraceptive used was included in family planning practices.

All these independent variables initially selected to predict RTI's are grouped according to the framework of determinants of reproductive morbidity proposed by Zurayk et al. (1993).

Biological susceptibility determinant
Presence of uterine with or without vaginal prolapse
Medical risk factor
Obstetric factors
Sterilization operation
Intermediate Determinants
Age
Personal Hygiene
Menstrual Practices and Hygiene
Awareness of RTI
Husband staying separately
Background Determinants
Economic condition
Relation of the women with the head of the household
Type of family
Education

Figure 7.1: RTI's and the Determinants

A. *Background Determinants of Reproductive Tract Infection*

Table 7.12: RTI and Background Determinants

Variable	*Total number of women*		*Prevalence of RTI*		*P-Value*	
	Andro (N=194)	*Kwakei-thel (N=190)*	*Andro (N=194) No. (%)*	*Kwakei-thel (N=190) No. (%)*	*Andro*	*Kwakei-thel*
Women's education					< 0.001	< 0.001
Illiterate	103	39	45 (43.7)	19 (48.7)		
Literate	91	151	8 (8.8)	16 (10.6)		
Total family income per month (Rs.)					< 0.05	< 0.01
1000-4000	152	47	48 (31.6)	17(35.4)		
5000-9000	35	61	5 (14.3)	16(26.2)		
10,000-14,000	0	30	0 (0)	2(6.9)		

Type of family						
Nuclear	140	137	30 (21.4)	5 (3.6)	< 0.004	< 0.001
Joint	53	53	23 (43.3)	30 (56.6)		
Relation of women with the head of the household						
Daughter-in-law	43	50	16 (37.2)	27 (54.0)		
Sister-in-law	10	4	6 (60.0)	4 (100)	< 0.009	< 0.001
Wife	141	136	31 (22.0)	4 (2.9)		

* at 5% level of significance

Background correlates:

The literacy rate of women in Kwakeithel (79.5 percent) is more than that of Andro (46.9 percent). There are large number of nuclear families both in Andro (72.2 percent) and Kwakeithel (72.1 percent). In case of joint family, both Andro and Kwakeithel have the same number of household i.e.53 household. A high prevalence of infections was observed among illiterate women in both Andro and Kwakeithel and shows statistically significant correlation. Higher rate was also observed among lower income group in both the areas. Among the respondent's, women staying in joint family as daughter-in-law and sister-in-law in relation to the head of the household had high infection rate in both Andro and Kwakeithel.

B. *Intermediate determinants of Reproductive Tract Infection*

Table 7.13: RTI with Awareness of RTI and Husband Staying Away

Variable	*Total number of women*		*Prevalence of RTI*		*P-Value*	
	Andro (N=194)	*Kwakeit-hel (N=190)*	*Andro (N=194) No. (%)*	*Kwakeit-hel (N=190) No. (%)*	*Andro*	*Kwakeithel*
Awareness of RTI						
Yes	35	113	15 (42.9)	6 (5.3)	< 0.02	< 0.01
No	159	7	38 (23.9)	29 (37.7)		

Variable	*Total number of women*		*Prevalence of RTI*		*P-Value*	
	Andro (N=194)	*Kwakeithel (N=190)*	*Andro (N=194) No. (%)*	*Kwakeithel (N=190) No. (%)*	*Andro*	*Kwakeithel*
Husband staying away					< .001	<0.001
Yes	12	23	11 (91.7)	18 (78.3)		
No	182	167	42 (23.1)	17 (10.2)		

* at 5% level of significance

As women are reluctant to talk about their individual sexual behaviour, a proxy variable was included in an attempt to measure a time period for which women and their husband's were separated because of work. This variable was found to be significantly associated with the presence of reproductive tract infections. In Andro, among those women whose husband stay away 91.7 percent were found having infection. In Kwakeithel, 78.3 percent were found having infection among women whose husband stay away.

Looking at the "degree of awareness" regarding reproductive tract infections women in Kwakeithel were more well aware about the disease related to it than the women in Andro. This is reflected in the number of women in Andro (18.0 percent) and Kwakeithel (59.4 percent) who are aware of reproductive tract infections. A higher prevalence of infection was observed amongst the women respondents who are not aware of reproductive tract infections in Kwakeithel (37.7 percent) while in Andro, the percentage is high among women who are aware of reproductive tract infections.

Personal hygiene

Table 7.14: Personal Hygiene and RTI

Variable	*Total number of women*		*Prevalence of RTI*		*P-Value*	
	Andro (N=194)	*Kwakeit-hel (N=190)*	*Andro (N=194) No. (%)*	*Kwakeit-hel (N=190) No. (%)*	*Andro*	*Kwakei-thel*
Take bath daily						
Yes	176	186	50(28.4)	18 978.3)	< 0.220	<0.001
No	18	4	3 (16.7)	17 (10.2)		
Place of bath						
Pond						
Common tap	33	4	11 (33.3)	9 (19.1)		
Common hand pump	11	72	4 (33.3)	12 (16.7)		
	46	71	12 (26.1)	14 (19.7)	< 0.84	<0.886
Just outside the hutment	102	0	26 (25.5)	0 (0)		
Wash private part						
Yes	105	127	3(2.9)	1 (0.8)	< 0.001	<0.001
No.	89	63	50 (56.2)	34 (54.0)		
Change undergarment						
Yes	0	105	0 (0)	4 (3.8)	< 0.001	<0.001
No	194	85	53 (100)	31 (23.1)		
Wash hand before eating						
Yes	34	105	0	4 (3.8)	< 0.001	<0.001
No	160	85	53 (33.1)	31 (36.5)		
Boil drinking water						
Yes	23	177	0	32 (18.1)	< 0.001	<0.665
No	171	13	53 (31.0)	3 (23.1)		
Wash hand after defecation						
Yes	34	106	0	32 (18.1)	< 0.001	<0.001
No	160	84	53 (33.1)	3 (23.1)		

* at 5% level of significance

Personal hygiene which includes washing of private parts, washing hands after defecation, taking bath daily, place of taking bath, etc. plays a pivotal role for a healthy reproductive tract. Due to lack of awareness about health and hygiene, a large number of women did not maintain personal hygiene in Andro. 45.9 percent of women in Andro did not wash their private parts while taking bath. Out of this 45.9 percent, 56.2 percent of women had infection which points towards the fact that women who do not wash their private parts have high chance of getting reproductive tract infection. In Kwakeithel, 33.2 percent of women did not wash their private parts while taking bath and among them 54.1 percent had infection in their reproductive tract. Besides this, personal hygiene like washing hand before having food, boiling of drinking water, washing of hand after defecation are found to be comparatively less in Andro than in Kwakeithel which shows that there is a need to educate women about the maintenance of personal hygiene. This variable was also significantly associated with the presence of Reproductive Tract Infections.

Menstrual hygiene

Table 7.15: RTI and Menstrual Hygiene

Variable	*Total number of women*		*Prevalence of RTI*		*P-Value*	
	Andro (N=194)	*Kwakeithel (N=190)*	*Andro (N=194) No. (%)*	*Kwakeithel (N=190) No. (%)*	*Andro*	*Kwakeithel*
Type of material used						
Phanek	49	50	12 (24.5)	13 (26.0)		
Cloth	145	88	41 (28.3)	22 (25.0)	< 0.607	<0.001
Sanitary napkin	0	52	0 (0)	0 (0)		
Sex during Menses						
Yes	21	2	6 (28.6)	0 (0)	< 0.892	<0.51
No	173	188	47 (47.2)	35 (18.6)		

Variable	*Total number of women*		*Prevalence of RTI*		*P-Value*	
	Andro (N=194)	*Kwakeit-hel (N=190)*	*Andro (N=194) No. (%)*	*Kwakeit-hel (N=190) No. (%)*	*Andro*	*Kwakei-thel*
No. of Clothes changed in first 2 days						
1	8	0	7 (87.5)	0 (0)		
2	144	84	42 (29.2)	32 (38.1)		
3	42	91	4 (9.5)	3 (3.3)	< 0.001	<0.001
4	0	13	0 (0)	0 (0)		
Wash private parts during menstruation						
Yes	0	146	0 (0)	3 (2.5)		<0.001
No	194	44	53 (27.3)	32 (72.7)		

* at 5% level of significance

Perineal hygiene like management of monthly period is another vital factor for a healthy reproductive tract. During menstruation, no women in Andro reported of washing their private parts. While in Kwakeithel, 23.1 percent of women did not wash their private parts. In Andro all the women who had infection was among those women who did not wash their private parts during menstruation. In Kwakeithel, among women who did not wash their private parts during menstruation, 72.7 percent of had reproductive tract infection.

Reproductive tract infections are also related to the type of soaking material used and the frequency of changing the soaking material during menstrual period. In Andro, none of the women had reported of using sanitary pad as soaking material. In Andro, 28.3 percent of women using cloth as soaking material had infection while in Kwakeithel 25.0 percent of the women using cloth had infection and shows statistically significant relationship.

The frequency of the soaking material and reproductive tract infections shows significant relationship. In Andro, 8 women use one pad a day in the first two days and among them, 87.5 percent had infection while women in Kwakeithel change twice or more. In Kwakeithel, 6.8 percent of the women reported of changing four times a day in the first two days. However, in Andro, none of the women reported of changing four times a day. In Andro, 21.6 percent of the women change thrice while in Kwakeithel, 47.9 percent of the women change the soaking material three times a day in the first two days. Thus, variance in the type of soaking material as well as in the frequency of changing the soaking material could be seen in Andro and Kwakeithel.

C. Medical Risk Factor

There is a positive association between women who have had invasive obstetric/gynecological procedure and abortion with reproductive tract infections. Women who have had undergone abortion had higher prevalence of infection in both Andro and Kwakeithel. In Andro out of the 36 women who had undergone abortion 61.1 percent were found infected in their reproductive tract. In Kwakeithel, 40.9 percent women were found having reproductive tract infections among 22 women who had undergone abortion.

Obstetric factor

Table 7.16: RTI and Obstetric Factors

Variable	*Total number of women*		*Prevalence of RTI*		*P-Value*	
	Andro (N=194)	*Kwakeit-hel (N=190)*	*Andro (N=194) No. (%)*	*Kwakeit-hel (N=190) No. (%)*	*Andro*	*Kwakei-thel*
Age at marriage						
15-19	60	0	17 (28.3)	0 (0)		
20-24	96	71	25 (26.0)	10 (14.1)	< .351	<0.272
25-29	30	86	11 (36.7)	20 (23.3)		
30-34	0	26	0 (0)	3 (11.5)		
35-39	0	4	0 (0)	2 (50.0)		

Variable	*Total number of women*		*Prevalence of RTI*		*P-Value*	
	Andro (N=194)	*Kwakeit-hel (N=190)*	*Andro (N=194) No. (%)*	*Kwakeit-hel (N=190) No. (%)*	*Andro*	*Kwakei-thel*
No. of living children						
≥ 2	72	95	21 (29.2)	16 (16.8)	< .660	<0.576
≤ 2	122	95	32 (26.2)	19 (20.0)		
Birth place of last baby						
Home	171	0	52 (30.4)	0 (0)	< .04	
Hospital	10	190	1 (10)	35 (18.4)		
Person attending the delivery						
Maibi	23	0	7 (30.4)	0 (0)		
Doctor	10	190	1(10)	35 (18.4)	< 0.119	
Nurse	148	0	45 (30.4)	0 (0)		
Material used for cutting the cord						
unsterilised blade	22	0	7 (31.8)	0 (0)	< 0.747	
sterilized blade	158	190	45 (28.5)	35 (18.4)		
Abortion/ stillbirth						
Yes	34	22	22 (64.7)	9 (40.9)	< 0.001	<0.004
No	160	168	31 (19.3)	26 (15.5)		
Place of abortion/ stillbirth						
Not applicable	160	168	41 (25.6)	26 (15.5)		
PHC	22	0	0 (0)	0 (0)		
Maibi's place	5	0	4 (18.2)	0 (0)	< 0.037	<0.04
Home	1	0	4 (66.7)	0 (0)		
Hospital	6	22	4 (80.0)	9 (40.9)		

Variable	*Total number of women*		*Prevalence of RTI*		*P-Value*	
	Andro (N=194)	*Kwakeit-hel (N=190)*	*Andro (N=194) No. (%)*	*Kwakeit-hel (N=190) No. (%)*	*Andro*	*Kwakei-thel*
Person attending the abortion/ stillbirth						
Not applicable	160	168	41 (25.6)	26 (15.5)		
Maibi	6	0	4 (66.7)	0 (0)		
Doctor	20	22	3 (15.0)	9 (40.9)	<0.01	<0.04
Nurse	8	0	5 (62.5)	0 (0)		
Contraceptive use						
None	89	54	21 (23.6)	5 (9.3)		
IUD	49	20	12 (24.5)	10 (50.0)		
Oral pill	31	14	10 (32.3)	4 (11.4)	< 0.398	<0.001
Sterilization	24	82	10 (41.7)	15 (19.0)		
Condom	0	20	0 (0)	1 (3.0)		

* at 5% level of significance

The place and person attending the abortion too plays a pivotal role. In Kwakeithel, abortions were conducted only in the hospitals by the doctors but in Andro, abortions were conducted by *maibi* at home, nurse at Primary Health Center and by the doctors at the hospitals/clinics in Imphal. A good percentage of women (66.7 percent) whose abortion was conducted by *maibi* at home had Reproductive Tract Infection.

In Andro, there is also high prevalence of reproductive tract infection among women who gave birth to the last baby at home either by a nurse or *maibi*. Out of the 23 women delivered by the *maibi* at home 7 were infected. Among the 148 deliveries done by the nurse at home 30.4 percent had Reproductive Tract Infections.

In Kwakeithel, women who had ever used an IUD or were currently using IUD, high prevalence of infections was observed and were found to be significantly associated with the presence of RTI. In Andro, high prevalence of infection was observed amongst those women who had undergone sterilization operation. The plausible explanation could be the fact that sterilization operations conducted under the government health system are often done in an unhygienic condition.

D. *Biological Susceptibility Determinants*

Table 7.17: RTI and Prolapse

Area	*Variable*	*Total number of women*	*Prevalence of RTI no. (%)*	*P-Value*
Andro	Prolapse			
(N=194)	Yes	52	21 (40.4)	< 0.013
	No	142	32 (22.5)	
Kwakeithel	Prolapse			
(N=190)	Yes	23	8(34.8)	< 0.031
	No	167	27 (16.2)	

* at 5% level of significance

Infections were higher among women who have genital prolapse in Andro thus indicating a significant correlation between prolapse and chance of getting infection. However, the scenario is different in Kwakeithel. As a biological susceptibility determinant, prolapse too showed association with RTI in Andro but not in Kwakeithel.The prevalence of infection is more among those women who did not had genital prolapse.

The salient features that have emerged up from the findings are that uneducated, poor women are mostly infected. Home deliveries and abortion conducted by untrained persons have higher frequency of infection. Sterilization operation in Andro and IUD user in Kwakeithel were significantly associated with the prevalence of reproductive tract infection.

E. *Determinants of Genital Prolapse*

Independent variables were selected to predict prolapse and are grouped in accordance to the framework developed by Zurayk et al. (1993). The risk factors were examined for the presence of at least one form of genital prolapse. The different forms of prolapse were pooled in. Data for the construction of background and intermediate determinants were obtained from survey form. In both Andro and Kwakeithel variables like age, type of family, women's position relative to other women in the household, parity and sterilization operation are included in the final model as they were significantly associated in prolapse in bivariate analysis. However, variables like income, stillbirth/abortion were found insignificant hence were not included in the final model.

A woman who had three or more deliveries had higher frequency of prolapse than those women who had two or less deliveries. Age is also another factor. In Andro, the number of women who had prolapse increases with the increase of age. However, in Kwakeithel, prolapse was found among women in 40's. Women who are in their 40's have higher prevalence of prolapse than those who are younger. Type of family and position of women in relation to other women in the household were found to be positively associated with the presence of genital prolapse. Income was also included, to check the possible relation with genital prolapse but was found insignificant.

Table 7.18: Genital Prolapse and Determinants

Variable	*Total number of women*		*Prevalence of Prolapse*		*P-Value*	
	Andro (N=194)	*Kwakeithel (N=190)*	*Andro (N=194) No. (%)*	*Kwakeithel (N=194) No. (%)*	*Andro*	*Kwakeithel*
Age (Years)						
25-29	35	0	1 (2.9)	0(0)		
30-34	43	0	5 (11.6)	0(0)		
35-39	48	0	13 (27.1)	0(0)	< 0.001	< 0.001
40-44	26	45	19 (73.1)	2(24.4)		
45-49	19	42	14 (73.7)	12(28.6)		
Education						
Illiterate	103	39	32 (31.1)	12 (30.8)	< 0.154	< 0.001
Literate	91	151	20 (22.0)	11 (7.3)		

Variable	*Total number of women*		*Prevalence of Prolapse*		*P-Value*	
	Andro (N=194)	*Kwakeit-hel (N=190)*	*Andro (N=194) No. (%)*	*Kwakeit-hel (N=194) No. (%)*	*Andro*	*Kwakeit-hel*
Income (Rs.)						
1000-4000	152	49	41 (27.0)	7 (14.3)		
5000-9000	32	63	9(28.1)	11 (17.5)		
10,000-14,000	7	29	1 (14.3)	3 (10.3)		
15,000-19,000	0	15	0 (0)	0 (0)	< 0.885	< 0.526
20,000-24,000	3	16	1 (33.3)	1 (6.3)		
25,000-29,000	0	9	0 (0)	0 (0)		
30,000-34,000	0	7	0 (0)	0 (0)		
50,000-54,000	0	2	0 (0)	1 (14.3)		
Type of family						
Nuclear	140	55	18 (12.9)	18 (32.7)	< 0.001	< 0.001
Joint	54	135	34 (63.0)	5 (3.7)		
Relation of the women with the head of the household						
Daughter-in-law	43	52	23 (53.5)	16 (30.8)		
Sister-in-law	10	4	10(100)	2 (50.0)	< 0.001	< 0.001
Wife	141	134	19 (13.5)	5 (3.7)		
No. of living children						
0-2	72	95	1 (1.4)	0 (0)	< 0.001	< 0.001
3-8	122	95	51 (41.87)	23 (24.2)		
Family Planning method						
Contra-ceptive	80	49	27 (33.8)	3 (6.1)	< 0.001	< 0.001
Operation	25	87	19 (76.0)	20 (23.0)		
None	89	54	6 (6.7)	0		

Variable	*Total number of women*		*Prevalence of Prolapse*		*P-Value*	
	Andro (N=194)	*Kwakeit-hel (N=190)*	*Andro (N=194) No. (%)*	*Kwakeit-hel (N=194) No. (%)*	*Andro*	*Kwakeit-hel*
Contra-ception used	89	54	6 (6.7)	0		
None	49	20	27 (55.1)	0		
IUD	31	20	0	3 (15.0)	< 0.001	< 0.001
Oral	1	14	0	0		
Vasectomy	25	3	19 (76.0)	0		
Tubectomy	0	79	0 (0)	20 (25.3)		
Condom						
Stillbirth / Abortion	36	22	10 (27.)	1 (4.5)	< 0.885	< 0.219
Yes	158	168	42 (26.6)	22 (13.1)		
No						

* at 5% level of significance

Intermediate Variable

Age

Parity

Sterilization operation

Background Variable

Type of family

Women's position in the household

Figure 7.2: Prolapse and Determinants

To surmise, age, type of family, women's position in relation to other women in the household, parity and sterilization are positive predictors of genital prolapse in both Andro and Kwakeithel.

To surmise, this chapter presents the data collected during clinical phase of the field work. The correlation of the clinical findings and the laboratory results of vaginal discharge and genital prolapse with the women's self reported symptoms of *phingou chatpa* as well as *angang khao nanthaba/hakchang mapan thokpa* are highlighted to understand the sensitivity of the signs and symptoms reported by women. The findings reflects that the degree of association between women's report of *phingou chatpa* with clinical and laboratory diagnosis of vaginal discharge is not good in both Andro and Kwakeithel. However, women's self reported symptoms of *angang khao nanthaba/hakchang mapan thokpa* with the clinical diagnosis of prolapse shows concordance and hence can be taken as a good predictor.

This chapter also accentuates the risk factors of Reproductive Tract Infections in both Andro and Kwakeithel constructing on the model founded by Zurayk. As a background co relate, socio-economic variables like education, type of family, relation of the women with the head of the household, family income per month are potent factors in both Andro and Kwakeithel for reproductive tract infections. Among the intermediate co relate, variables like awareness of reproductive tract infections, husband staying away once in a month, personal hygiene and menstrual hygiene are taken up and are found to be statistically significantly. Among the medical risk factors, sterilization and obstetric factors were found to be significantly co-related with the presence of reproductive tract infections. From the findings, it can be concluded that Kwakeithel women are more aware of reproductive tract infections, perineal hygiene as well as about the management of menstrual hygiene.

8

Implication of Reproductive Health on Policy and Programme

This chapter endeavors to bridge the gap between what we think is the need (top down) and what is the actual need at the grassroots level (felt need). It is a brain storming pedagogic exercise to address the reproductive health problem in Andro and Kwakeithel as well as provide a basis of recommendation to health and family planning providers.

This anthropological and epidemiological exploration of reproductive health of women underscores the need to incorporate women's perception of their bodies and the practices they follow with these beliefs to design an implication of health programme as well as provide a basis of recommendation to health and family planning providers. Beliefs and cultural perspectives affect people in both overt and subtle ways on their attitude towards illness. Meanings are embodied in the term "illness" and symptoms are filtered through the worldview of the people. The incorporation of women's perception of their illness at the backdrop of their beliefs and practices will endeavour to facilitate in designing a culturally sensitive programme. The entry point could be the identification, prevention and mitigation of harmful beliefs and practices simultaneously promoting positive ones.

8.1 WOMEN'S BELIEFS AND PRACTICES

Women's ethno-anatomy and ethno-physiology of both Andro and Kwakeithel succinctly differs from the bio-medically derived anatomical models, both spatially and functionally. Women describe the body part as they feel and experience them, not having an opportunity to "look inside" a body. They describe the body parts which could be physically felt from outside and which women feel through experience of body processes like pregnancy. Beliefs about a variety of physiological processes: menstruation, conception, sexual behaviour and childbirth practice associated with these beliefs provide insights into potential determinants of reproductive illness.

8.1.1 Menstruation:

During menstruation, woman is considered impure and therefore polluting, a finding which is prevalent throughout India (Nichter, 1981). In accordance with this belief, women follow menstrual practices which may be unhygienic and therefore a risk factor for reproductive tract infections (Younis et al., 1993). Women said that they do not take bath until their menstrual flow ceases for fear of polluting their surrounding raising concerns about menstrual hygiene. Bivariate analysis also shows significant relationship between women who do not wash their private parts during menstruation and the prevalence of reproductive tract infections in both Andro and Kwakeithel. In Kwakeithel, 72.7 percent of the women who do not wash their private parts during menstruation had infection while in Andro none of the women reported washing their private part during menstruation and all the women who had infection (53) did not wash their private parts during menstruation.

Another cause of concern is the lack of awareness of healthy perineal hygiene practices and the belief that wearing panties will obstruct the flow of the blood in Andro. In this regard, women in Kwakeithel have better knowledge and awareness about menstrual hygiene than their counterpart in Andro which is reflected in the data of soaking material used by them and also the frequency of changing the soaking material. In Andro, none of the women reported using sanitary napkin, 74.7 percent used old or any piece of clothes and 25.2 percent of women use phanek as soaking material during menstruation. In Kwakeithel, 26.3 percent of women use phanek, 46.3 percent use clothes and 30.5 percent use sanitary napkin as the soaking material. In Andro, among women who wore phanek during menstruation, 24.5 percent were infected and 28.3 percent of women who use clothes had infection while in Kwakeithel, none of the women who use sanitary napkin were found having infection, 26 percent of the women who wore phanek had infection and 25 percent of the women who use clothes were found having infection.

The frequency of changing clothes in the first two days shows significant relationship with infection, 87.5 percent of women who change once in the first two days were infected. The number of infected women decreases with the increase in frequency of changing the clothes/pads in the first two days. Maintenance of perineal hygiene is of importance in the prevention and control of reproductive tract infections (Garg et al., 2000). The present study also indicates that the use of hygienic practices for the perineum like usingnapkin and washed clothes during menstrual period was found among educated women in Andro and Kwakeithel. However, the fact that many women in Andro and some women in Kwakeithel were found using unclean *phanek* and old clothes for the perineal hygiene reflects ignorance, unaffordability of napkins due to poverty as well as the need to hide menstruation due to social practices. The use of unwashed *phanek,* old clothes or any other clothes by women in Andro and Kwakeithel for maintaining perineal hygiene in greater frequency requires adequate intervention and education in disinfecting the *phanek,* clothes which could be done by washing, boiling and drying under the sun. It also calls for the need to organize awareness campaigns in the study areas so that women can adopt healthy perineal hygienic practices in the community.

8.1.2 Conception:

Women in Andro and Kwakeithel perceive that a child is conceived when a man's *mahik* (germ) meet the woman's blood. This perception suggests that women link menstruation with conception and this can be used in controlling fertility.

8.1.3 Sexual Behaviour:

Women's perception about their sexual functions was informative for several reasons. Issues relating to sexual and reproductive health are often highly sensitive and even tabooed to discuss openly in both the areas though there is some relaxation in Kwakeithel. Often the language of sex is an area of contention. Taboo and silence limits the possibilities of opening spaces for people to be able to express themselves and share their experiences. The belief and practices that illnesses concerning women's reproductive health are considered as shameful and women suffering from such ailments are stigmatized and marginalized. Such an attitude has resulted in women being reluctant to discuss the situation or to seek health care. Complications due to fear of reprimandation hovers around.

Education can help the women in opening up the mindset and improving awareness of and encouraging appropriate health seeking behaviour could potentially alleviate such contentions. The belief that illness can be communicated from man who sleeps with another woman and the disapprovement of extra marital sexual encounter is one positive strategy in preventing reproductive tract infections.

Beliefs and practices of sexual abstinence during menstruation and childbirth were reported by women in this study. Women believe that sexual intercourse during this period will lead to illness. These beliefs and practices may serve as an effective entry point through which family planning strategies may be introduced.

8.1.4 Childbirth:

Women's belief and practices regarding childbirth provide vital information about the risk factors for infection or prolapse associated with childbirth. Description of the delivery practices in Andro such as the insertion of fingers into the cervix and pulling the fetus out during a hard labour reveal the possibility of risk factor of infection and prolapse that are associated with childbirth.

The belief of cutting the umbilical cord with *wakthou* (a kind of bamboo) so that the child will grow tall and sturdy like the bamboo tree can be risky as it is not sterilized. Bivariate analysis also shows significant relationship of infection with the cutting of chord with unsterilized material.

30.4 percent of women who gave birth at home by *maibi* (traditional birth attendant)/nurse were infected in Andro. While only 10 percent of women who gave birth at the hospital were infected. 31.8 percent of deliveries where unsterilized blade/ *wakthou* was used for cutting cord were infected. In Andro, delivery where sterilized blades was used 28.5 percent were infected while in Kwakeithel 18.4 percent were infected.

8.1.5 Women's Illness:

Women refer to health problems relating to reproductive organs and functions not as "reproductive" illnesses but as *nupigi anaba* (women's illness). They perceive that *anangba* (poverty) is the root cause of *nupigi anaba* (women's illness). Conditions directly resulting from *anangba* (poverty) include anger, worry, lack of nutritious food and hard toil. These conditions will in turn produce *sonthaba* (physiological weakness) which makes a woman vulnerable to illnesses associated with sterilization operation, copper-T use, abortion, delivery problems, lifting heavy weights and sexual intercourse.

Women visualize "women's illnesses" as the outcome of successive stages of weakening of which the root cause is poverty. Furthermore, the result shows that women associate weakening phenomena such as menstruation, childbirth and the ability to provide sufficient nutrition to women throughout their life cycle with the fact that they are women, therefore, resulting in "women's illnesses".

The findings from the comparison of women's self reported symptoms of *phingou chatpa* and *angang khao nanthaba/hakchang mapan thokpa* with the clinical examination of vaginal discharge and laboratory result has far reaching implication for the treatment of reproductive tract infections based on reports of vaginal discharge as recommended by WHO. *Phingou chatpa* was found to be a moderate predictor of vaginal discharge in Andro (66.3 percent) and Kwakeithel (54.4 percent) and poor predictor of clinically diagnosed reproductive tract infection in Andro (38.5 percent) and Kwakeithel (44.3 percent). The laboratory diagnosed vaginitis also shows low predictive value of 35.6 percent in Andro and 43.6 percent in Kwakeithel with low level of agreement assessed by Kappa correlation in Andro raging from 0.5 to 0.05 and moderate level of agreement (Kappa=0.4 to 0.5).

Table 8.1: Comparison of Women's Self Reported Symptom with Diagnosis based on Clinical and Laboratory Findings

Women's self report or clinical examination	*Area*	*Sensitivity (%)*	*Specificity (%)*	*PPV (%)*	*NPV (%)*	*Agreement (%)*	*Kappa*	*Clinical observation/laboratory diag-nosis*
Phingou chatpa	Andro	48.1	92.3	69.4	82.9	94	0.83	Discharge
	Kwakeithel	95.6	96.4	78.5	99.3	96	0.82	
Phingou chatpa	Andro	83.3	56.1	38.5	91.1	62.9	0.29	Clinical vaginitis/ cervicitis
	Kwakeithel	100	76.6	44.3	100	76.8	0.48	

Women's self report or clinical examination	*Area*	*Sensitivity (%)*	*Specificity (%)*	*PPV (%)*	*NPV (%)*	*Agreement (%)*	*Kappa*	*Clinical observation/laboratory diag-nosis*
Phingou chatpa	Andro	80	55.2	35.6	89.9	61.1	0.247	Laboratory vaginitis
	Kwakeithel	100	71.2	43.6	100	76.5	0.474	
Angang khao nanthaba/ hakchang mapan thokpa	Andro	48.1	92.3	69.4	82.9	94	0.83	Prolapse
	Kwakeithel	95.6	96.4	78.5	99.3	96	0.82	

Table 8.2: Comparison of Clinical Vaginitis/Cervicitis with Laboratory Vaginitis

clinical examination	*Area*	*Sensitivity (%)*	*Specificity (%)*	*PPV (%)*	*NPV (%)*	*Agreement (%)*	*Kappa*	*laboratory diagnosis*
Clinical vaginitis/ cervicitis	Andro	100	97.9	93.8	100	98.4	0.056	Laboratory vaginitis
	Kwak-eithel	100	99.3	97.1	98.1	99.4	0.98	

The above results suggest the possibility that women might report *phingou chatpa* as a symptom which doesn't mean vaginal discharge to them but is used to describe other phenomena. This possibility was also suggested by results of the Egypt study (Zurayk et al., 1995) that demonstrate high sensitivity for a complaint of discharge but low predictive value and poor agreement with medically diagnosed reproductive tract infections. Zurayk et al., have suggested that women's perceived morbidity has an impact on reported morbidity.

The ethno-medical model constructed on women's perception of illness will be useful for an analysis of the perceived determinants of gynecological morbidity and health seeking behavior.

Women articulate poverty as the single most important cause of their illnesses. Women perceive "women illnesses" as a "semantic" network of physical, mental and emotional states. They perceive that physical problems like weakness; discharge, menstrual problems along with or as a consequence of emotional, mental states of anxiety, worry and anger all within the context of poverty.

To illuminate the situation, mention can be made of the Bryon Good's "semantic" analysis of illness in his discussion of "heart distress", an Iranian folk illness (Good, 1977). The theoretical basis of such an analytical framework lies in the concept that illness categories may be understood as a "syndrome of experiences" and as a core of a semantic network of feelings, situations and symptoms (Good, 1977) all joined together in a polysemic relationship, were polysemy is defined as "the property of a symbol to relate to a multiple range of symbols" (James Fox, 1975 cited in Good, 1977).

I propose that the category of illness described by the term *phingou chapta* is related to feelings, physical symptoms and situations in a network of meanings and that different meaning are socially generated by individuals to articulate their experience. The ethnographic findings show that *phingou chapta* is used interchangeably with other physical symptoms such as weakness. Additionally women describe the feeling of impoverishment, anger and anxiety in connection with *phingou chatpa*. Pachauri and Gittelsohn (1994) also reported of association between discharge and other physical symptom, although they suggested that terms like weakness was used euphemistically for discharge. Nichter (1981) in his study among South Indian women about the idioms of psychosocial distress found that women using "illness idiom", among other idiom of purity, devotion, spirit, food to express their distress. Illnesses mentioned by women who visited a traditional healer includes discharge, menstrual complaints, weakness, digestive disorders, overheat, back and body pain among other complaints. On further examination, Nichter found that women either reported discharge directly or with related terms like weakness and were experiencing stressful situation in their lives; women complained of discord in their families such as conflict with their mother-in-law, sexual tension with their husband and economic problem in the household (Nichter, 1981).

Oomman (1996) in her work among the rural Rajasthan women recognized the importance of studying the cultural meaning of words such as "weakness" when used to describe gynecological problems. Her findings explicate that women's report of *dhola pani* do not map with bio-medically defined disease categories. She found that women in rural Rajasthan associate poverty as the cause of illness and therefore an underlying synergism of poverty and pathology. Oomman concludes that reproductive tract infections represent 'disease" a pathological state while *dhola pani* represents "illness" a condition of impoverishment (Oomman, 1996).

Results from this study also exhibit similar findings. Women's perception of their bodies and illness give us an insight of their impoverished life and demonstrates the distress which women express as illness, which is interchangeably used as weakening too. However, such a model does not deny the fact that a large proportion of women who had reported of *phingou chatpa* actually have vaginal discharge. Instead, it provides an explanation for one of the many reasons of discordance between women's report of *phingou chatpa* and medically diagnosed reproductive tract infections.

The comparison of women's report of *angangkhaonanthaba/hakchang mapan thokpa* show high predictive value in Andro (69.4 percent) and Kwakeithel (78.5 percent) and high degree of agreement in both the areas with Kappa of 0.83 and 0.82 in Andro and Kwakeithel. These results show that reported system of prolapse is a good predictor for the presence of prolapse.

This study proposes that symptom reporting is a dynamic process, resulting from interaction between perceived morbidity and the situation in which a woman reports a symptom. Thus, an illness is the meaning that individual give to health and refers to a person's perception and experiences of certain socially disvalued states. The meaning of health needs to be recognized for achieving an analytical understanding of the process of production of health as a basis for any realistic and comprehensive effort to improve health condition in the community. Women's health behaviour, particularly seeking health care is also governed by what women perceived as ill health.

In Andro and Kwakeithel women's perception of *anangba* (poverty) as the root cause of illnesses can be one big factor in restraining women from seeking health care. Women unanimously believe that improvement of their impoverished life will prevent them from being weak and therefore less vulnerable to women's illnesses. Conditions directly resulting from poverty include anger, anxiety, lack of food to eat and hard toil. These conditions result in *sonthaba* (weakness) which makes a woman susceptible to illnesses associated with sterilization operation, copper-T use, abortion, delivery problems and lifting heavy weights. Since the women perceive that their illnesses are due to poverty and not due to biomedical cause, they will not participate in gynecological clinics. This can corroborate with evidence from the percentage of women who did not seek any treatment.

Majority of women in both Andro and Kwakeithel did not seek any treatment for all the three illnesses. In Andro, 98.1 percent of women having menstrual problem 53.7 percent of women having vaginal discharge and91.7 of percent of women suffering from prolapse did not take any treatment. In Kwakeithel 82.1 percent of women having menstrual problem, 52.7 percent of women having vaginal discharge problem and 18.9 percent of women suffering from prolapse did not seek treatment. Though the percentage of women who did not seek treatment for menstrual problem and prolapse in Kwakeithel are comparatively less, the percentage of women suffering from vaginal discharge who did not seek treatment is high in both Andro and Kwakeithel. The plausible reason can be the belief that poverty is the root cause of illnesses and that alleviation of their impoverished life will improve their health condition.

Another possible reason for not taking any treatment for illness is the distance of the health provider from the area where they live. In Andro, the number of women suffering from prolapse who did not undertake any treatment is 91.7 percent, which is high. Women in Andro believe that prolapse can be cured only by undergoing operation and the Primary Health Center which is the nearest health care center in Andro does not have adequate infrastructure and facilities to conduct such kind of surgical procedures. For treatment of prolapse, they have to go to the hospital in Imphal. Andro is 26 kilometers away from Imphal. A woman has to traverse this distance by bus. The bus will terminate in one corner of Imphal and from the bus terminal she has to take a rickshaw to reach the hospital. It consumes time as well as money. Lack of money to cover the cost of transportation and treatment refrained women from seeking treatment. Thus, distance also limits women's willingness and ability to seek care. Bringing service closer to women-through provision of mobile service would overcome many of the distance and transport constrains currently affecting access to care.

Another main approach which can be made is towards enhancing the informative base of women for better care, hygienic practices, maintenance and management of menstruation especially in rural Andro.Due to lack of awareness about health and hygiene, a large number of women did not maintain personal hygiene in Andro. 45.9 percent of women in Andro did not wash their private parts while taking bath. Out of this 45.9 percent, 56.2 percent of women had infection which points towards the fact that women who do not wash their private parts have high chance of getting Reproductive Tract infection. In Kwakeithel, 33.2 percent of women did not wash their private parts while taking bath and among them 54.1 percent had infection in their reproductive tract. Besides this, personal hygiene like washing hand before having food, boiling of drinking water, washing of hand after defecation are found to be comparatively less in Andro than in Kwakeithel which shows that there is a need to educate women about the maintenance of personal hygiene. This variable was also significantly associated with the presence of Reproductive Tract Infections.

Another finding is that there is statistically significant relationship in the prevalence of infection and women who had undergone sterilization operation or women who are currently using intra uterine device. About 41.7 percent of women in Andro and 19 percent of women in Kwakeithel who have undergone sterilization operation have at least one reproductive tract infection or another. One plausible explanation could be fact that sterilization operations which were conducted under the government health system were unhygienic. Other studies have also examined the positive association between contraception use and reproductive tract infections in developing countries (Wasserheit et al., 1981, Younis et al., 1993, Oomman., 1996) focusing on intra uterine device use.

A hospital based study in India has suggested a positive association between sterilization operation and infection (Kochar, 1985). Another clinic based study showed that tubectomized women in Bangladesh were seven times more likely to have an infection than women who had not been tubectomized (Wasserheit et al., 1989). The finding that sterilized women are twice as likely to have reproductive tract infection compared to unsterilized women should be considered in light of the fact that since 1983, over four million female sterilization operations are performed annually in India. This makes the possibility of iatrogenic infection due to sterilization a concern in terms of the disease burden it might cause for rural Indian women. (Brabin et al., 1992).

The findings from the study show the difference in the percentage of women who had undergone sterilization and the prevalence of reproductive tract infection in Kwakeithel and Andro. The case in Andro is more than in Kwakeithel. This explicates the unhygienic condition of conducting sterilization operation in rural areas. This finding provides a basis for recommendation to health and family planning providers. The risk of infection from laparscopy may be circumvented to prevent reproductive morbidities especially since contraceptive associated risk for infection is influenced by government policy. The government can mandate and check that all laparoscopic operation are conducted hygienically and provide a wider choice of safe contraception.

To surmise, this chapter provides a basis for recommendation to the government policy and programme. It underscores the need to incorporate women's perception of their bodies its function and illnesses. The incorporation of women's perception of their illness at the backdrop of their belief and practices will facilitate in designing a culturally sensitive programme. This is essential as women's perception of illness do not map with the bio-medically defined disease. The study findings also exudates the need to educate women regarding about menstrual hygiene and practices. An awareness programme on clean surrounding and healthy existence is a must.

Lastly, it is the government's duty to mandate and check that all laparoscopic operation are conducted hygienically and provide a wider choice for safe contraception and provisions to bring service closer to women in rural areas.

9
Conclusion

The title of this book accentuates the reproductive health of women in Andro and Kwakeithel. The write up begins with why study of women's reproductive health is the need at this hour. The inscription also highlight the rich tapestry of life in Andro and Kwakeithel- the *pana* institution in Andro which is the learning center about their ancestry, ritual, customs and the festivals which insinuate an unstinting devotion on supernatural being. It also essayed on the surroundings, means of communication, health care facilities, etc.

This work was embarked on the premises that ill health should be explored both as a "disease" as well as an "illness". This book progressed from a description of women's cultural construction of their bodies and illness culminating in an ethno-medical model of illness to compare women's reported symptom and clinical diagnosis of gynecological morbidity, and finally to determine the predictors of the two main locally perceived health problem, reproductive tract infection and prolapse.

Women in rural Andro and peri-urban Kwakeithel have their own distinct cultural construction of their body parts and its function. Women's ethno-anatomy and ethno-physiology succinctly differ from the biomedically derived anatomical models both spatially and functionally. They describe body parts as they feel and experience them not having an opportunity to "look inside" the body. They describe the body parts which could be felt from outside and which women feel through experience of body processes like pregnancy. However, women were able to describe some internal organs of the body and their function in coherent fashion.

This perception of body parts by women will serve as a backdrop of their perception of "women's illnesses".

Certain hazardous beliefs and practices which jeopardize the reproductive tract are also highlighted in this study. Harmful menstrual belief and practices like not taking bath during menstruation for fear of polluting the surrounding with menstrual blood is a cause of concern as it infects reproductive tract. Menstrual hygienewhich includes the type of soaking material used, washing of private parts during menstruation and number of clothes changed in the first two days was found to be statistically significant with infection. In Andro, among women who wore *phanek* during menstruation, 24.5 percent were infected and 28.3 percent of women who use clothes had infection while in Kwakeithel, none of the women who use sanitary napkin were found having infection. Here 26 percent of the women who wear *phanek* had infection and 25 percent of the women who use clothes were found having infection.

In Andro, none of the women reported using sanitary napkin, 74.7 percent used old or any piece of clothes and 25.2 percent of women use *phanek* as soaking material during menstruation. In Kwakeithel, 26.3 percent of women use *phanek*, 46.3 percent use clothes and 30.5 percent use sanitary napkin as the soaking material.

The frequency of changing clothes in the first two days also showed significant association with infection, 87.5 percent of women who change once in the first two days in Andro were infected. The number of infected women decreased with the increase in frequency of changing the clothes/ pads in the first two days.

Women's belief and practices regarding childbirth provide vital information about the risk factors for infection or prolapse associated with childbirth. Description of the delivery practices in Andro such as the insertion of fingers into the cervix and pulling a foetus out during labour reveal the possibility of risk factor of infection and prolapse that are associated with childbirth.

The belief of cutting the umbilical cord with *wakthou* (a kind of bamboo) so that the child will grow tall and sturdy like the bamboo tree can be risky as it is not sterilized. Bivariate analysis also shows significant relationship of infection with the cutting of cord with unsterilized material.High prevalence of reproductive tract infection among women who deliver their babies at home by the *maibi*/nurse is observed in rural Andro with an unsterilized blade/*wakthou.* 30.4 percent of women who gave birth at home by *maibi*/nurse were infected in Andro while only 10 percent of women who gave birth at the hospital were infected. 31.8 percent of delivery where unsterilized blade/*wakthou* was used for cutting cord resulted in infection. In Andro, delivery where sterilized blades was used, 28.5 percent were infected while in Kwakeithel 18.4 percent were infected.

These cultural belief and practices can be prevented or mitigated to reduce the infection of reproductive tract in Andro. On the other hand belief and practices of sexual abstinence during menstruation and childbirth may serve as an effective entry point through which family planning strategies can be introduced.

Women in both rural Andro and peri urban Kwakeithel self reported at least one symptom prior to the clinical examination. The frequency of most commonly reported symptoms namely *Phingou chatpa* (vaginal discharge), *mangbaga mari leinaba anaba* (menstrual problem) and *angang khao nanthaba/ hakchang mapan thokpa* (prolapse) were more in Andro than in Kwakeithel. Symptoms of digestive problem, circulatory/respiratory, infertility and weakness (exhaustion) problem during intercourse were reported more in Kwakeithel than in Andro.

Check listing of selected illness increases the magnitude of reporting the problem. After prompting, problem during intercourse increased by 50 percent in Andro and 38.4 percent in Kwakeithel. The higher percentage in Andro suggested that women in Andro are more conservative in their outlook than their counterpart in Kwakeithel. Women in Kwakeithel are more educated and are more open in their outlook. The fact is that women remain silent and bear the brunt of illness because of fear of being stigmatized or encroaching tabooed topic. There is a need to make the women aware on the consequences and effect of hiding and prolonging such illnesses. Education will encourage women to open up their mindset. Among all the illness reported prior to the clinical examination, three main illnesses were chosen for this study based on the following criteria:

1. Most frequently mentioned in the free listing results.
2. Perceived that many women experience the illness.

3. An illness which women are hesitant to report because of the stigma associated with it and has been unattended to by health providers

The results of clinical examination revealed a high level of gynecological morbidity in Andro than in Kwakeithel. 35.6 percent of women in Andro were found having at least one gynecological morbidity, while Kwakeithel accounts for 27.9 percent. Women having two or more gynecological morbidity in Andro also outnumber women having two or more gynecological morbidity in Kwakeithel. In Kwakeithel, the frequency of women with no gynecological morbidity was 53.2 percent which is more than Andro. In Andro, clinical examination as well as laboratory results shows that 23.2 percent of women had vaginitis. In Kwakeithel, on clinical examination, 17.4 percent of women were found having vaginitis. When examined using laboratory method, 17.9 percent of women were found to have vaginitis. Laboratory assessment of the individual vaginal infection shows 7.7 percent and 6.3 percent of women having candidiasis in Andro and Kwakeithel. 13.7 percent and 9.5 percent of women had bacterial vaginosis while 2.6 percent and 2.1 percent of women were found to have trichomoniasis in Andro and Kwakeithel.

In Andro, 10.3 percent i.e. 20 women were identified having PID while in Kwakeithel only 2.6 percent i.e. 5 women were diagnosed having PID. It is hypothesized that PID may be prevalent in women due to previous lower reproductive tract and/or as infections which may be introduced through procedures like childbirth, abortion and sterilization operation.

Cervical screening is an important parameter of reproductive health. Clinically, cervical erosion was detected in 6.7 percent (13) of women in Andro and among 4.7 percent (9) women in Kwakeithel. The gynaecologist diagnosed a woman with cervical ectopy only when she observed an ectopy on the cervix where the squamous epithelium is replaced by columnar epithelium and has a bright red, clearly defined area on the vaginal aspect of the cervix. 13.4 percent of women were found to be clinically positive for cervicitis in Andro while in Kwakeithel 10.0 percent of women were detected having cervicitis. This explicates a better reproduction health condition among women in Kwakeithel than in Andro.

The prevalence of genital prolapse is more among women in Andro than the women in Kwakeithel, 26.8 percent and 12.1 percent of women in Andro and Kwakeithel showed at least one type of genital prolapse. 2.6 percent and 1.6 percent of women in Andro and Kwakeithel respectively had uterine prolapse only. 1.5 percent and 4.6 percent of women in Andro had only rectocoele and cystocoele. In Kwakeithel, the prevalence of only rectocoele and cystocoele was 0.5 percent. 4.1 percent in Andro and 0.5 percent of women in Kwakeithel were detected having cystocoele (anterior vaginal prolapse) and a uterine prolapse. In Andro, 4.6 percent of women and 2.6 percent of women in Kwakeithel had cystocoele, rectocoele and uterine prolapse.

During clinical examination, 25.8 percent of women were found to be free from gynecological morbidities in Andro. In Kwakeithel, the frequency of women with no gynecological morbidities was 53.2 percent which is comparatively high. 35.6 percent and 27.9 percent of women in Andro and Kwakeithel had one morbidity followed by women having two morbidities which are 26.8 percent and 15.8 percent, respectively in Andro and Kwakeithel. 8.8 percent and 1.1 percent of women in Andro and Kwakeithel had three morbidities. 2.1 percent and 1.0 percent of women in Andro were diagnosed having four and five gynecological morbidities while 1.1 percent were found having four and five gynecological morbidity in Kwakeithel.

The prevalence of high reproductive morbidity in Andro than in Kwakeithel may be due to two factors - rural and peri-urban environment and awareness of health. In rural Andro the health care facilities are not easily available. The village women have to cover a long way to Imphal (26 kms. away) to seek treatment which involves money and time. This compels them "not to take any action" for the treatment. In the case of Kwakeithel, many private clinics and government hospitals are within a furlong. In terms of time and availability of facilities women in Kwakeithel are in a better position than women in Andro. However, in both the areas, health seeking behavior pattern shows that most of the women did not take any treatment. Lack of awareness about the disease also slows down in taking up any action. Looking at the "degree of awareness" women in peri-urban Kwakeithel is more aware about the reproductive tract infection and the symptoms related to it than their counterpart in rural Andro. Education has helped women in Kwakeithel to be aware about the reproductive tract infections and related symptoms.

Women do not visualize health problems related to reproductive organs and functions as reproductive illness but they referred these illnesses as "*nupigi anaba*" (women's illnesses). An ethno-medical model of "women's illnesses" is the outcome from the women's perception of illness characteristics and etiology. This model suggests a linear mode of illness causation. Based on a linear model, it appears that women articulate *anangba* (poverty) as the root cause of illness. Conditions directly resulting from poverty include hard labour to make both ends meet and inability to afford to have nutritious food. These in turn produce *sothaba (*physiological weakness) which makes a woman susceptible to illnesses associated with sterilization operations, copper-T use, abortions, delivery problems, sexual intercourse and lifting heavy weights. The resulting common illnesses are *phingou chatpa* (vaginal discharge), *mangbaga mari leinaba anaba* (menstrual problem) and *angang khao nanthaba/hakchang mapan thokpa* (prolapse). Through women do not have a "germ theory" of illness they have a sense of illness pathology which is reflected in the above mentioned factor.

The aforementioned factors can be one of the potent reasons for the moderate concordance in the evaluation of women's reports with clinical observation and laboratory diagnosis. The evaluation of women's report of *phingou chatpa* with the clinical diagnosis and laboratory results indicate high sensitivity in both Andro and Kwakeithel which exhibits that women's reported the presence of *phingou chatpa* in the presence of high level of discharge and the presence of infection. However, moderate positive predictive value and moderate agreement of the term *phingou chatpa* indicates poor concordance between women's report with clinical and laboratory diagnosis. The moderate level of specificity indicates that a large number of women reported *phingou chatpa* when they have no discharge at all, no clinically and laboratory diagnosed infection. This could be attributed to the following : –

(i) Women have cleaned themselves prior to the gynecological examination removing any discharge that may have been present.

(ii) Women have misunderstood the question and have reported the post episode of *phingou chatpa*

(iii) Women have reported *phingou chatpa* as an illness which does not mean discharge to them.

Illness described by the term *phingou chatpa* is related to physical symptoms and situations in a network of meanings and different meanings are socially generated by individual to articulate their experiences. Results from the ethnographic phase of this study show that *phingou chatpa* is used with other physical symptom such as weakness. Additionally, this study found that women describe the feeling of impoverishment in connection with *phingou chatpa*. In other words, woman might report *phingou chatpa* if she is impoverished and feels weak although she might not have the physical symptom of vaginal discharge or if she has normal physiological discharge.

This shows that symptom reporting is a dynamic process resulting from an interaction between perceived morbidity and the situation in which a woman report a symptom. This, an illness is the meaning that women give to health and refers to a person's perception and experiences of certain socially disvalued status. The meaning of health needs to be recognized for achieving an analytical understanding of the process of production of health as a basis for any realistic and comprehensive effort to improve health condition in the community, as it has a direct bearing on the treatment seeking behavior. Thus, it underscores the need to incorporate women's perception of their illness in the light of women's belief about their bodies to design a culturally sensitive implication of health programs as well as provide a basis of recommendation to health and family planning providers.

Majority of women in both rural Andro and peri urban Kwakeithel did not seek any treatment. 98.1 percent and 82.1 percent of women having menstrual problem in Andro and Kwakeithel did not take any treatment. 53.7 percent of women in Andro and 52.7 percent of women in Kwakeithel having vaginal discharge did not seek any treatment. In Andro, 91.7 percent of women suffering from prolapse did not take treatment while in Kwakeithel 18 percent of women suffering from prolapse did not seek treatment.

One plausible explanation is the articulation of poverty as the root cause of illness by the women. This refrained woman from seeking health care. Women believe that alleviation of their impoverished life will improve their health condition hence, illness remain unattended.

Another constraining factor in seeking health are in rural Andro is distance. Distance of the health care center from the village limits women's willingness and ability to seek care. Financial constraint is another important factor in seeking timely care. The stigma attached to these illnesses which are remotely connected with reproductive health is another major hindrance to women seeking care.

The background determinants of reproductive tract infections showed that the prevalence of infections were high among illiterate women. The number of illiterate women in Andro is more than those in Kwakeithel. The high rate of infection was also observed among the lower income group women. The other risk factors which were found to be significant are: personal hygienewhich includes washing of private parts while taking bath, changing of undergarment if not taken bath, washing hands before eating, washing hands after defecation and boiling of drinking water. Women in Kwakeithel are more aware about self care activities like maintenance of personal hygiene and management of menstrual hygiene than their counterparts in Andro.

The proxy variable, which was included in this studying in an attempt to find husband's sexual behavior by measuring the time period for which women and their husband were separated because of work, was found significant in both the areas. This is one of the limitations of this study. Men's sexual behavior, their sex related illness and men's perception of women's illness has not been explored in this study to understand holistically men's role in the transmission of infection to women.

The medical risk factor which includes delivering of babies, abortion, sterilization operation, type of material used for cutting chord are also found to be significantly associated with the prevalence of reproductive tract infections.

Women also had undergone abortion conducted by a *maibi* is also another variable which is closely linked with reproductive tract infections. 66.7 percent of women whose abortion was conducted by a *maibi* had infection in Andro.

Another finding is that there is statistically significant relationship in the prevalence of infection and women who had undergone sterilization operation or women who are currently using intra-uterine device. 41.7

percent of women in Andro and 19.0 percent of women in Kwakeithel who had undergone such procedures reported at least one reproductive tract infection. This explicates the unhygienic condition of conducting sterilization operation in rural areas. This finding provides a basis for recommendation to health and family planning providers. The risk of infection from laparoscopy can be circumvented to prevent reproductive morbidities especially since contraceptive associated risks for infection is influenced by the government policy. The government can mandate and check that all laparoscopic operation are conducted hygienically and provide a wider choice of contraception.

Women's report of *angang khao nanthaba/hakchang mapanthokpa* with the clinical diagnosis of prolapse shows high agreement and therefore is a good predictor. The low sensitivity was attributed to women having vaginal prolapse who were not able to report it as it is neither visible nor felt by them. The remaining women did not report it as they were embarrassed to report it due to stigma attached to prolapse. The determinants of genital prolpase which are found to be statistically significant are age, number of children, type of family and relation of women with the head of the household.

This anthropological and epidemiological exploration of reproductive health of women underscores the need to incorporate women's perception of their illness in the light of women's belief about their bodies and the practice they follow with these belief to design a culturally sensitive implication of reproductive health programs as well as provide a basis of recommendation to health and family planning providers the "felt need" of the women. The entry point could be the identification, prevention and mitigation of harmful beliefs and practices simultaneously promoting positive ones.

A culturally sensitive program is a must as women's report of *phingou chatpa* do not go in congruence with the clinical and laboratory diagnosis of vaginal discharge. The finding explicates the underlying synergism of poverty and pathology which distinguishes "illness" from "disease". The thesis concludes that reproductive tract infection represent "disease" a pathological state while *phingou chatpa* represents "illness" a condition of impoverishment, emphasizing that one cannot be understood without the other. Therefore, there is a need to address the perceived "root cause" of their illness i.e. poverty to ameliorate the health condition of women in Andro and Kwakeithel. The time has come to look at the "felt needs" of the reproductive health of women. All human being have the basic right to a life free from hunger, poverty, ignorance, disease and fear.

There is also a need to create innovative health program which provides men and women with the knowledge to understand the "pathology" of disease within the context of their lives. There is a call for an approach towards enhancing the informative base of women for better care, hygienic practices, maintenance and management of menstruation especially in rural Andro.

To conclude, incorporation of women's perception of illnesses is essential to improve and make the reproductive health strategies more meaningful and relevant to the women in these two communities. Hope is the quintessence so, hope floats.

Bibliography

Adetunju, Jacob, A. (1996): Preserving the Pot and Water: A Traditional Concept of Reproductions Health in a Yoruba Community, Nigeria, *Social Science and Medicine*, 43 (11): 1561-67.

Adler, M.W. (1996): Sexually Transmitted Diseases Control in Developing Countries, *Genito Urinary Medicine*, 72: 83-88.

Agarwal, B., Bare, T.D., Henriques, M.L., Mathews, I., Chainery- Hesse, M., Ariffin, J., Ghaid, D., Jolly, R., Mc. Askie, C. And F. Stewart. (1990): *Engendering Adjustment for the 1990's: Report of a Commonwealth Expert Groups on Women and Structural Adjustment*, Commonwealth Secretariat: London.

Aggarwal A.K., Kumar, R., Gupta, V., Sharma, M. (1999): Community based Study of Reproductive Tract Infections among Ever-Married Women of Reproductive Age in a Rural Area of Haryana, India, *J. Commun. Disease*, 31:223-228.

AIDS, India (2006) Available in www.avert.org accessed Feb 1 2006.

Altman, D.G. (1991): *Practical Statistics for Medical Research*, Chapman and Hall: London.

Aral, S.O. and J. Wasserheit. (1998): Social and Behavioural Correlates of Pelvic Inflammatory Diseases, *Sexually Transmitted Diseases*, 25 (7): 378-85.

Baer, H.A., Singer, M., Susser, I. (1997): *Medical Anthropology and the World System: A Critical Prospective*, Beagin and Garvey: Westport.

Bahadur, M. and Santabi, Y. (1989): *Tribal Art of Manipur*, Mutua Museum: Imphal.

Bandarage, A. (1997): *Women, Population and Global Crises: A Political– Economic Analysis*, Zed Books: London.

Bang R. And Bang A.T (1994): Women's Perceptions of White Vaginal Discharge: Ethnographic Data from Rural Maharashtra. In Gittelsohn, J., Bentley, M.E., et al. (ed.) (1994): *Listening To Women Talk about their Health: Issues and Evidence from India,* Ford Foundation, Har-Anand Publications: New Delhi.

Bang, R.A. and Bang, A.T. (1992): Reproductive Tract Infections (RTI's): Rural Women's Point of View, *Manushi, a Journal about Women and Society,* 69:27-30.

Bang, R.A. and Bang, A.T. (1996): A Community Study of Gynecological Disease in Indian Villages: Some Experiences and Reflections, In S. Zeidenstein and K.Moore, (ed.): *Learning about Sexuality,* 223-237, the Population Council: New York.

Bang, R.A., Bang, A. Baitule, M., Chaudhary, Y., Sarmukaddam, S., and Tale, O. (1989): High Prevalence of Gynaecological Diseases in Rural Indian Women, *The Lancet,* 1(8629): 85-87.

Batliwala, S., Chitnis, S. and Fazalbhoy, N. (ed.) (1988): *The Health Status of Indian Women: a Reader,* Unit of Women's Studies, Tata Institute of Social Science: Bombay.

Bauman, D.B. (2003). A Rhetoric and Reality, *National Journal,* 35 (31): 2470-2476.

Beckmann, C.R.B. et al. (1992): *Obstetrics and Gynecology for Medical Students,* Williams and Wilkins: Baltimore.

Bennett. L. (1989): *Gender and Poverty in India: Issues and Opportunities Concerning Women in the Indian Economy,* World Bank Internal Document.

Berg, B.L. (1998): *Qualitative Research Methods for the Social Science,* Allyn and Bacon: Washington. Bernard H.R. (1988): *Research Methods in Cultural Anthropology,* Sage Publications: Newbury Park, CA.

Bernard, H.R., Pelto, P.J. et al. (1986): The Construction of Primary Data in Cultural Anthropology, *Current Anthropology,* 27(4): 382-396.

Bhatia J.C. and Cleland, J. (1996): Obstetric Morbidity in South India: Results from a Community Survey, *Social Science and Medicine,* 43: 1507-16.

Bhatia, J.C. and Cleland, J. (1995): Self-Reported Symptoms of Gynecological Morbidity and their Treatment in South India, *Studies in Family Planning,* 26(4): 203-216.

Bhatia, J.C. and Cleland, J., Bhagwan, L., and Rao, N.S.N. (1997): Levels and

Determinants of Gynecological Morbidity in a District of South India, *Studies in Family Planning*, 28(2): 95-103.

Bhatia, J.C. and Cleland, J. (1999): Health Seeking Behaviour of Women and Cost Incurred: An Analysis of Prospective Data, In Pachauri S. and Subramanium, S. (ed.): *Implementing a Reproductive Health Agenda in India: The Beginning*, The Population Council: New Delhi, 207-32.

Bhattacharya, M. (1963): *Gazzetter of India Manipur*, Anushilan Press: Calcutta.

Bhatti, L.I. And Fikree, F.F. (2002): Health Seeking Behaviours of Karachi Women with Reproductive Tract Infections, *Social Science and Medicine*, 54:105-117.

Bird, S.T., Bauman, K.E. (1995): The Relationship between Structural and Health Services Variables and State Level Infant Mortality in the United States, *American Journal of Public Health*, 85 (1):26-32.

Bongaarts, J. (1978): A Framework for Analyzing The Proximate Determinants Of Fertility, *Population Development Review*, 4(1): 105-132.

Boonmongkon, P. (2001): *Mot Luuk* Problems in North East Thailand, Why Women's own Health Concerns Matter as Much as Disease Rates, *Social Science and Medicine*, 53:1095-1112

Boonmongkon, P., Nichter, M., Pylypa, J., And Chantapasa, K. (1998): *Understanding Women's Experience of Gynecological Problems: an Ethnographic Case Study from Northeast Thailand*, Centre for Health Policy Studies, Mahidol University: Nakornpathom, Thailand.

Boserup, E. (1970): *Women's Role in Economic Development*, St. Martin's Press: New York.

Brabin, L., Kemp, J., Obunge, O.K., et al. (1995): Reproductive Tract Infections and Abortion among Adolescent Girls in Rural Nigeria, *the Lancet*, 3455(8945): 300-304.

Bulut, A., Yolsal, N., Fillippi, V., and Graham, W. (1995): In Search of Truth: Comparing Alternative Sources of Information on Reproductive Tract Infection, *Reproductive Health Matters*, No. 6, November.

Campbell, O. and Graham, W. (1990): *Measuring Maternal Mortality and Morbidity: Levels and Trends. Maternal and Child Epidemiological Unit*, London School of Hygiene and Tropical Medicine: London.

Census of India. (2001): Primary Census Abstract available from www. censusindia.net Accessed March 1.2005.

Centers for Disease Control (CDC) Staff and Outside Experts, (1991): Pelvic Inflammatory Disease: Guidelines for Prevention and Management, *Morbidity and Mortality Weekly Report,* 40(RR-5): 1-25.

Central Bureau of Health Intelligence. (2003): Health Information of India, DGHS,

Government of India: Delhi

Chatterjee, M. (1991): *Indian Women: Their Health and Productivity,* World Bank Discussion, Paper 109, World Bank: Washington, D.C.

Chatterjee, M. (1991): *Towards Better Health for Indian Women. The Dimensions, Determinants and Consequences of Female Illness and Death,* Paper Prepared for The World Bank Economic Sector Work on Women and Health.

Cladwell, J. And Cladwell, P. (1991): What Have we Learnt about the Cultural, Social And Behavioural Determinants of Health?, *Health Transition Review* 1(1):13-19.

Clifford, J. And Marcus, G.E. (ed.) (1990): *Writing Culture: The Poetics and Politics of Ethnography,* Oxford University Press: Delhi.

Cliquet, R., and Thienpont, K. (1995): *Population and Development: A Message from the Cairo Conference,* Kluwer: Dordrecht.

Correa, S., and Reichmann, R.L. (1994): *Population and Reproductive Rights: Feminist Perspectives from the South,* Zed Books: London.

Davis, K. and Blake, J. (1956): Social Structure and Fertility: An Analytical Framework, *Economic Development and Cultural Change,* 4:211-235 .De Vellis, R.F. (1991): *Scale Development: Theory And Applications,* Applied Social Research Methods Series, Sage Publications, Newbury Park.

Dixon –Mueller, R. (1993): "Population Controllers" And the Feminist Critique, In *Population Policy and Women's Rights: Transforming Reproductive Choice,* 31-54 Praeger: West Port.

Dixon- Mueller, R. and Wasserheit, J. (1991): *The Culture of Silence: Reproductive Tract Infection among Women in the Third World,* International Women's Health Coalition: New York.

Dixon–Mueller, R. (1993): The Sexuality Connection in Reproductive Health, *Studies in Family Planning,* 24 (5): 269-282.

Dodson, M.G. and Faro, S. (1985): The Polymicrobial Etiology of Acute Pelvic Inflammatory Disease and Treatment Regimens, *Review of Infectious Diseases,* 7(4): 696-702.

Duley, M.I. and Edwards, M.I. (ed.) (1986): *The Cross Cultural Study of Women: A Comprehensive Guide*. The Feminist Press: New York.

Elias, C. (1996): *Infection free Sex and Reproductive Health, Reproductive Health in Developing Countries: Expanding Dimensions, Building Solutions*, National Academi Press: Washington, D.C.

Eschenbach, D.A. (1980): Epidemiology and Diagnosis of Acute PID, *Obstetrics and Gynecology*, 55:142-153.

Eschenbach, D.A. (1993): Bacterial Vaginosis and Anaerobes in Obstetric-Gynecologic Infection, *Clinical Infectious Diseases*, 16 (4): 282-287.

Fabrega, H. (1972): The Study of Disease in Relation to Culture, *Bahavioural Science*, 17:183-203.

Fathalla, M, (1991): Reproductive Health: A Global Overview, *Annals of the New York Academy of Sciences*, 626:1-10.

Finger, W.R. (1992): What Should You Know about STDS?, *Network* ,12 (4) 2-3.

Frakenberg, R. (1980) Medical Anthropology and Development: A Theoretical Perspective, *Social Science and Medicine*, 14 B: 197-207.

Gandhi, N., And Shah, N. (1993): *The Issues at Stake: Theory and Practice in the Contemporary Women's Movement in India*, Kali for Women: New Delhi.

Garg, S., Sharma, N., Sahay, R., Bhalla P. (2000): *An Epidemiological and Sociological Study of Symptomatic and Asymptomatic Reproductive Tract Infections among Women in an Urban Slum*, Task Force Project Report, Department of Community Medicine, Maulana Azad Medical College: New Delhi.

George, A., Shah, I., and Nandraj, S. (1994): *A Study of Household Health: Expenditure in Madhya Pradesh*. Foundation for a Research in Community Health: Mumbai.

Germain, A. (1987): *Reproductive Health*'s *And Dignity: Choices By Third World Women*, Technical Background Paper Prepared For The International Conference On "Better Health For Women and Children through Family Planning", Nairobi, Kenya. International Women's Health Coalition: New York.

Germain, A. and Kyte, R. (1995): *The Cairo Consensus: the Right Agenda for the Right Time*, International Women's Health Coalition: New York.

Germain, A., Holmes, K.K., Piot, P. and Wasserheit, J.N. (ed.). (1992): *Reproductive Tract Infection: Global Impact and Priorities for Women's Reproductive Health*, Plenum: Press: New York.

Germain, A., Holmes, K.K., Piot, P., And Wasserheit, J.N. (1992): *Reproductive Trait Infectious: Global Impact and Priorities for Women's Reproductive Health,* Plenum Press: New York.

Gittelsohn, J., Bentley, M.E., et al. (ed.) (1994): *Listening to Women talk about their Health: Issues and Evidence from India,* Har-Anand Publications: New Delhi.

Gittelsohn, J., Pelto, P., Bentley, M., Nag, M. and Oomman, N. (1994): Qualitative Methodological Approaches for Investigating Women's Health in India, In Gittelsohn, J., Bentley, M.E., et al. (eds.) (1994): *Listening to Women Talk About their Health: Issues and Evidence from India,* Har-Anand Publications: New Delhi.

Gogate, A., Brabin, S., Nicholas, S., Gogate, T., Goankar, A., Naidu, A., Divekar, A., Karande and Hart G.A. (1998): Risk Factor for Laparoscopically Confirmed Pelvic Inflammatory Disease. Findings from Mumbai (Bombay), India, *Sexually Transmitted Infections,* 74: 4216-32.

Good B.J. (1977): The Heart of What's the Matter: The Semantics of Illness in Iran, *Culture, Medicine and Psychiatry,* 1:25-58.

Grierson, G.A. (1967): *Linguistics Survey of India,* Vol. I. Part I., Motilal Banarasidass: Delhi.

Hammond, Dorothy and Jablow. (1976): *Women in Culture of the World,* Cummings Publishing Company: New York.

Heaver, R., (1992): Participatory Rural Appraisal: Potential Applications in Family Planning, Health and Nutrition Programmes, In *Special Issue on Applications for Health, RRA Notes,* Number 16, International Institute For Environment And Development: London.

Helman, C.G. (1990): *Culture, Health and Illness: An Introduction for Health Professionals,* Wright: London.

Hudson, T.C. (1975): *The Meithei's,* Low Price Publication: Delhi

Honingmann, J.J. (1959): *The World of Man,* Harper and Bro.Pub: New York.

Ibungohal, L. (1987): *Introduction to Manipur,* the Saraswati Printing Works: Imphal.

Imoba, Rabikanta and Rajketan. (1999): *Pottery in Manipur,* Mutua Museum: Imphal.

International Institute for Population Sciences (IIPS). (1995): *National Family Health Survey (NFHS): India 1992-1993,* IIPS, Bombay.

Ismail, S.O. (1990): Syphilis, Gonoerhoea and Genital Chlamydia Infection in a Somali Village, *Genito Urinary Medicine*, 6670-75.

Jacobson, J.L. (1991): *Women's Reproductive Health: the Silent Emergency*, Worldwatch Paper 102, Worldwatch Institute: Washington, D.C.

Jeffery, P., Jeffery, R., Lyon, A. (1989): *Labour Pains and Labour Power: Women and Childbearing in India*, Zed Publishers: London.

Jejecbhoy, S. and M Koenig. (2002): The Social Context of Gynecological Morbidity, In S. Jejeebhoy, M.Koenig and C.Elias (ed.): *Research Approaches To The Study Of Reproductive Tract Infections and Other Gynecological Disorders*, Cambridge University Press: Cambridge.

Jossens, M.O. and Sweet, R.L. (1993): Pelvic Inflammatory Disease: Risk Factors and Microbial Etiologies, *JOGNN*, March/ April: 169-177.

Kaddour, A., Hajez, R., Zurayk, H., (2005): Women's Perceptions of Reproductive Health in Three Communities around Beirut, Lebanon, *Reproductive Health Matters*, 13 (25): 34-42.

Kanani, S., Latha, K., Shah, M. (1994): Application of Qualitative Methodologies to Investigate Perceptions of Women and Health Practitioners Regarding Women's Health Disorders in Baroda Slums, In Gittelsohn, J., Bentley, M.E.., et al. (ed.) (1994): *Listening To Women Talk About Their Health: Issues and Evidence from India*, Ford Foundation, Har-Anand Publication, New Delhi.

Kraal, M., Gupta, M. and Sadgopal, M. (1995): Women, Health and Development, *Radical Journal of Health: A Socialist Health Review Trust Publication, Bombay*, 1:25-36.

Khanna, J. (2001): *Progress in Reproductive Health Research*, UNDP/UNFPA/ WHO/World Bank Special Programme on Research, Development and Research Training in Human Reproduction, WHO: Geneva, Switzerland.

Kitzinger, J. (1995): Introducing Focus Groups, *British Medical Journal*, 317: 299-302.

Kleinman, A. (1997): *Writing at the Margin: Discourse between Anthropology and Medicine*, University of California Press: Berkely.

Kleinman, A., (1980): *Patients and Healers in the Context of Culture: An Exploration of the Borderland between Anthropology, Medicine and Psychiatry*, University of California Press: Berkeley.

Kleinman, A., Eisenberg, L. and Good, B. (1978): Culture, Illness and Care:

Clinical Lessons from Anthropologic and Cross-Cultural Research, *Annals of Internal Medicine,* 88:251-258.

Kochar, M. (1980): Etiology of Pelvic Infections Treated by Gynecologic Service of the Kasturba Hospital, Delhi, India, *American Journal of Obstetric and Gynecology,* 138:872-874.

Koenig, M., Jejeebhoy, S., Singh, S., Sridhar, S. (1998): Investigation Women's Gynecological Morbidity in India not just another KAP Survey, *Reproductive Health Matters,* 6 (11): 84-97.

Laga, M. (1992): "Human Immunodeficiency Virus Infection Prevention: The Need for Complementary Sexually Transmitted Disease Control". In A. Germain, K.K Holmes, P. Piot, And J.N. Wasserheit (ed.): *Reproduction Tract Infection; Global Impact and Priorities for Women's Reproduction Health,* Plenum Press: New York and London, 131-144.

Lane, S.D. and Meleis, A.I. (1991): Roles, Work, Health Perceptions and Health Resources of Women: A Study in an Egyptian Delta Hamlet, *Social Science and Medicine,* 33(10):1197-1208.

Latha K.,Kanani, S.J.,Maitra, N.,Bhatt, G.B., Senapati S.K., Bhattacharya, S.,Sridhar, S.,Giri, G.B.,Shah,P.P.,Shah, S.P.,Desai, L.A., Parikh, I.,Taskar,V., Dharap, N.,Mulgaonkar,V. (1997): Prevalence of Clinically Detectable Gynecological Morbidity in India: Results of Four Community Based Studies, *The Journal of Family Welfare,* 43(4):8-16.

Luthra, U.K., Mehta, S., Bhargava, N.C., Ramchandran, P., Murthy, N.S., and Sexena, B.N. (1992) Reproduction Tract Infections in India: The Need for Comprehension Reproductive Health Policy and Programme, In A Germain, K.K. Holmes, P. Piot and J.N. Wasserheit.1992. *Reproductive Tract Infections: Global Impact and Priorities for Women's Reproductive Health,* Plenum Press: New York.

Luthra, U.K., Mehta, S., Ramachandran, P., Murthy, N.S., Seghal, A., and Saxena, B.N. (1992): Reproductive Tract Infections in India: The Need for Comprehensive Reproductive Health Policy and Programs, In Germain A., et al. (ed.) (1992): *Reproductive Tract Infections: Global Impact and Priorities for Women's Reproductive Health,* Plenum: New York.

Mac Cormack, C. (1985): Lay Concepts Affecting Utilization of Family Planning Services in Jamaica, *Journal of Tropical Medicine and Hygiene,* 88:281-285.

Mac Cormack, C.P. (ed.) (1982): *Ethnography of Fertility and Birth,* Academic Press: London.

Manipur State AIDS Control Society. (2004): "Status Report of National AIDS Control Programme 2003-2004", Manipur, Imphal.

Mardh, P.A. (1980): An Overview of Infection Agents in Salpingitis: Their Biology And Recent Advances in Methods of Detection, *American Journal of Obstetrics and Gynecology*, 138:933-51.

Mc Carthy, J. And Maine, D. (1992): A Framework for Analyzing the Determinants of Maternal Mortality, Implications for Research and Programs, *Studies in Family Planning*, 23(1): 23-33.

McElroy, A. and Townsend, P.K. (1989): *Medical Anthropology in Ecological Perspective*, Westview Press: Boulder.

Measham, A. and Heaven, M. (1995): *India's Family Welfare Program: Moving to a Reproductive and Child Health Approach, Directions is Development*, World Bank: Washington D.C., USA.

Ministry of Health and Family Welfare, Family Welfare Programme in India (2003): Department Of Family Welfare: New Delhi

Mishler, E.G. (1981): Viewpoint: Critical, Perspectives on the Biomedical Model, In Mishler, E.G. (ed.): *Social Contexts of Health, Illness and Patient Care*, Cambridge University Press: Cambridge.

Mosha. F., Nicholl, A. et al. (1993): A Population Based Study of Syphilis and Sexually Transmitted Disease Syndromes in North Western Tanzania: Prevalence and Incidence, *Genitourinary Medicine*, 69:425-420.

Mosley, W.H. and Chen, L. (1984): An Analytical Framework for the Study of Child Survival in Developing Countries, In Mosley, W.H., And Chen, L. (ed.) *Child Survival: Strategies for Research, Population Development Review*, 10:25-45.

Mueller, D.R., and Wasserheit, O. (1991): *The Culture of Silence: Reproductive Tract Infections among Women in the Third World*, International Women's Health Coalition: New York.

Mulgoankar, V.B., Parikh, I.G., Taskar, V.R. et al. (1994): Perceptions of Bombay Slum Women Regarding Refusal to Participate in a Gynecological Health Programme, In Gittelsohn, J., Bentley, M.E. et al. (ed.) (1994): *Listening to Women Talk about their Health: Issues and Evidence from India*, Har-Anand Publications: New Delhi.

NACO Country Scenario 1998-1999; National AIDS Control Organisation, Ministry of Health and Family Welfare, Government of India.

Nag, M. (1993): Consultant Trip Report Submitted to the Project, *Building Social Science Research for Women's Reproductive Health in India,* Consultant Trip Report Submitted to the Ford Foundation, India.

Naorem, S. (ed.) (1988): *Manipur: Past and Present,* Vol.I, Mittal Publication: Delhi.

Narayan, N. and Srinivasan, S. (1994): Some Experiences in the Rapid Assessment of Women's Perceptions of Illness in Rural and Urban Areas of Tamil Nadu, In Gittelsohn, J. Bentley, M.E., et al. (ed.) (1994): *Listening to Women Talk about their Health: Issues and Evidence from India,* Har-Anand Publications: New Delhi.

National Family Health Survey-2 (1992-93): International Institute of Population Sciences, Mumbai 2000.

Nations, M.K. (1986). Epidemiological Research on Infectious Diseases: Quantitative Rigor or Rigormortis? Insights from Ethnomedicine, In C.R. Janes, R. Stall and S.M. Gifford (ed.): *Anthropology and Epidemiology: Interdisciplinary Approaches to the Study of Health and Disease,* 97-123, Dordrecht: Reidel.

Nichter, M. (1981): Idioms of Distress: Alternatives in the Expression of Psychosocial Distress: A Case Study from South India, *Culture, Medicine and Psychiatry,* 5:379-408.

Norren, B. and Vianen, H. (1986): *The Malnutrition. Infections Syndrome and its Demographic Outcome in Developing Countries,* PCDO/ Programming Committee for Demographic Research: The Hague.

Obeyesekere, G. (1976): The Impact of Ayurvedic Ideas on the Culture and the Individual in Sri Lank, In C. Leslie, (ed.): *Asian Medical Systems: A Comparative Study,* University of California Press: Berkeley.

Oomman, N.M. (1996): *Poverty and Pathology: Comparing Rural Rajasthani Women's Ethnomedical Models with Biomedical Model of Reproductive Behaviour,* Ph.D. Thesis, Johns Hopkins University: Baltimore, Maryland.

Ortner, S.B. (1974): Is Female to Male as Nature is to Culture? In Rosaldo and Lamphere, (ed.) *Women, Culture and Society,* Stanford University Press: Palo Alto.

Pachauri, S. (1994): Relationship between AIDS and Family Planning Programmes: A Rationale for Development Integrated Reproductive Health Services, *Health Transition Review,* 4 Suppl: 321-47.

Pachauri, S. and Gittelsohn, J. (1994): Summary of Research Studies and Implications for Health Policy and Programmes, In Gittelsohn, J., Bentley, M.E., et al. (ed.) (1994): *Listening To Women Talk about their Health: Issues and Evidence from India,* Har-Anand Publications: New Delhi.

Padian, N., Shiboski, S.C. and Hitchcock, P.J. (1991): Risk Factors for Acquisition of Sexually Transmitted Diseases and Development of Complication, In J. Wasserheit, S.O. Aral, K.K. Holmes and P.J. Hitchcock (ed.): *Research Issues in Human Behaviour and Sexually Transmitted Diseases in the AIDS Era,* American Society For Microbiology: Washington, D.C.

Patel, B.C., Barge, S., Kothe, R. and Sadhwani, H. (1994): Listening to Women Talk about Their Reproductive Health Problems in the Urban Slums and Rural Areas of Baroda, In Gittlelsohn, J., Bentley, M.E., et al. (ed.) (1994): *Listening to Women Talk about their Health: Issues and Evidence from India,* Ford Foundation, Har-Anand Publications: New Delhi.

Patel, T., (1994): *Fertility Behaviour: Population and Society in A Rajasthani Village,* Oxford University Press: Delhi, India.

Ramasubban, R. (1996): Patriarchy and The Risk of STD and HIV Transmission to Women, In M. Das Gupta, L. Chen and T. N. Krishnan (ed.): *Women's Health in India. Risks and Vulnerability,* 213-241, Oxford University Press: Oxford.

Registrar General of India, Census of India, Series–1, (2000): India. Provisional Population Tables, Paper–1 of 2001, Controller of Publications: New Delhi.

Registrar General of India. (2000): Sample Registration System, Statistical Report.

Rosaldo, M.Z. and Lamphere, L. (ed.) (1974): *Woman, Culture and Society,* Stanford University Press: CA.

Ross, J.A. (1998): *The Policy Project Targets for Family Planning in India: An Analysis of Policy Change, Consequence and Alternative Choices.* The Futures Group: New Delhi, India.

Sanday, P., (1974) In Rosaldo, M.Z. And Lamphere, L. (Eds.) (1974): *Woman, Culture and Society,* Stanford University Press: CA.

SEWA Rural Research Team, (1994): Beliefs and Behaviour Regarding Diet During Pregnancy in a Rural Area in Gujarat, Western India, In Gittelsohn, J., Bentley, M.E. et al (ed.) (1994): *Listening to Women Talk about their Health: Issues and Evidence from India,* Har-Anand Publications: New Delhi.

Shenoy, K.T., Shenoy, S., Gopalakrishnan, K., (1997): *Reproductive Health and Gynecological Morbidity in Kerala*, Draft Report.

Shorter, F. (1987): *The Production of Health in Cairo Households*, Paper Presented at the Population Council Workshop on Assessment of Health Interventions, Cairo.

Singer, M., (1989): The Limitations of Medical Ecology: The Concept of Adaptation in the Context of Social Stratification and Social Transformation, *Medical Anthropology*, 10:223-234.

Singh, M.M., Joshi, P.C., Sapir, D.G., Marx, M., Picquet, M., Thakur, J.S., Mukherjee, B.M., Saklani, B., Bapna, J.S., Roy, P. (2003): *Self-reported symptoms of reproductive tract infections among ever-married women aged 15-40 years: a multi centric study*. 47th National Conference of Indian Public Health Association, Nagpur, Maharashtra state, India, 17-19th January.

Singh, M.M., Joshi, P.C., Sapir, D. G., Marx, M., Roy, P., Bapna, J.S. (2002): Utilization of health care services in relation to diarrhoeal disease, mental illness and women's reproductive health problems in rural Alwar, Rajasthan, 29th Annual Conference of Indian Association of Preventive and Social Medicine, Wardha, 15-17th February.

Singh, S. (1995): *Three Year Sting at Sonagachi: An Exposition, The STD/HIV Intervention Programme at Sonagachi, 1992-95*, All India Institute of Hygiene and Public Health: Calcutta, India

Spradley, J.P. (1979): *The Ethnographic Interview*, Holt, Rinchart and Winston, Inc.: Chicago.

Stamm. W.E. et al. (1988): *The Practitioner Handbook for the Management of STD's*, Health Sciences Center for Educational Resources: University of Washington, USA.

Talaat, M., Watts, S., Mekheimar, S., Ali, H.F., Hamed.H. (2004): The Social Context of Reproductive Health in an Egyptian Hamlet: A Pilot Study to Identify Female Genital Schistosomiasis, *Social Science and Medicine*, 58: 515-524.

Temmerman et al. (1998): The Supermarket for Women's Reproductive Health: The Burden of Genital Infections in a Family Planning Clinic in Nairobi, Kenya, *Sexually Transmitted Infections*, 74:202-204.

Thaddeus, Serene and Maine, D. (1990): *Too Far To Walk: Maternal Mortality in Context*, Prevention of Maternal Mortality Program, Center for Population and Family Health: Columbia University.

Tindall, I. (ed.) (1990): *Persistent Inequalities: Women and Third World Development*, Oxford University Press: New York.

United Nation. (1995): Summary of the Program of Action of the International Conference on Population and Development, 1994, 13, New York, United Nation.

United Nations. (1994): Report of the International Conference on Population and Development, Cairo, September 5-13.A/CONF.

Wasserheit, J.N. (1989): The Significance and Scope of Reproduction Tract Infections among Third World Women, *International Journal of Gynecology and Obstetrics*, Suppl. 3: 145-68.

Wasserheit, J.N. (1989): The Significance and Scope of Reproductive Tract Infections among Third World Women, *International Journal of Gynecology and Obstetrics*, Suppl. 3:145-68.

Wasserheit, J.N. (1990) Reproductive Tract Infections, In *Special Challenges in Third World Women's Health*, Presentations to The 117th Annual Meeting of The American Public Health Association in Chicago, Illinois, International Women's Health Coalition: New York.

Wasserheit, J.N. and Holmes, K.K. (1992): Reproductive Tract Infections: Challenges for International Health Policy, Programs and Research, In German A. et al. (ed.) (1992): *Reproductive Tract Infections: Global Impact and Priorities for Women's Reproductive Health*, Plenum Press: New York.

Wasserheit, J.N., Harris, J.R., et al. (1989): Reproductive Tract Infections in a Family Planning Population in Rural Bangladesh, *Studies in Family Planning*, 20(2): 69-80.

Weller, S.C. and Romney, A.K. (1990): *Systematic Data Collection*, Sage Publications India Pvt. Ltd.: New Delhi.

Westrom, L. and Mardh, P. (1975): Acute Salpingitis: Aspects of Aetiology, Diagnosis and Prognosis, In Daniellson, D., Juhlin, L. et al. (ed.): *Genital Infections and Their Complications*, Almqvist and Wiksell International: Stockholm.

Whittaker, A. (1996): White Blood and Falling Womb: Ethnogynecology in Northeast Thailand. In P.L. Rice and L. Manderson (ed.): *Maternity and Reproductive Health in Asian Societies*, Harwood Academic Publishers: Amsterdam.

Winikoff, B. (1988): Women's Health-An Alternative Perspective for Choosing Interventions, *Studies in Family Planning*, 19(4): 197-214.

World Health Organization. (1995): *Sexually Transmitted Diseases : Three Hundred and Thirty-Three Million New, Curable Cases in 1995,* Press Release, WHO/64, August 25, 1995.

World Health Organization. (1996): A Reproductive Health Approach to a Safer Motherhood.

Young, A. (1982): The Anthropologies of Illness and Sickness, *Annual Review of Anthropology,* 11:257-285.

Young, J.C. (1981): *Medical Choice in a Mexican Village,* Rutgers University Press: New Jersey.

Young, P.V. (1966): *Scientific Social Surveys and Research,* Prentice-Hall of India Private Limited: New Delhi.

Younis, N., Khattab H, Zurayk H., Et Al. (1993): A Community Study of Gynecological and Related Morbidities in Rural Egypt, *Studies in Family Planning,* 24(3): 175-186.

Younis, N., Khattab, H., Zurayk, H., et al. (1993): A Community Study of Gynecological and Related Morbidities in Rural Egypt, *Studies in Family Planning,* 24(3): 175-186.

Zurayak, H. Khattab, H., Younis, N., et al. (1995): Comparing Women's Report with Medical Diagnosis of Reproduction Mobility in Rural Egypt, *Studies in Family Planning* , 26 (1):14-21.

Zurayk, H., Khattab, H., Younis, N., El-Mouelhy, M., (1993): Concepts and Measures of Reproductive Morbidities in Rural Egypt, Studies in Family Planning, 3 (1):17-40.

Index

N

O

P

R

S

T